15-Day Herbal Gut Reset

Break Free from Failed Detoxes and Reclaim Your Digestive Health

Mary B. Hubb

Table of Contents

Dedication

To my family and friends, for your unwavering support, patience, and love throughout this journey.

To those seeking a path to healing and well-being—may this book inspire you to take control of your health and embrace the power of nature.

Acknowledgments

This book would not have been possible without the guidance, encouragement, and wisdom of many people along the way. I am deeply grateful to all those who contributed to the creation of The 15-Day Herbal Gut Reset.

To my mentors and colleagues in the health and wellness community—thank you for your inspiration and the knowledge you've shared with me. Your work has motivated me to explore natural remedies and embrace holistic healing.

I also want to express my gratitude to my friends and family, who provided endless encouragement, understanding, and love throughout this process. You've been my rock, and I couldn't have done this without you.

Finally, to my readers—thank you for trusting me as a guide on your path to better health. I hope this book empowers you to break free from failed detoxes and reclaim your digestive health, one step at a time.

With gratitude,

Mary B. Hubbs

Introduction

Overview of Gut Cleanse's Benefits

Cleansing the gut has become a popular practice for improving overall health, boosting energy levels, and promoting better digestion. The human gut is home to trillions of microorganisms, collectively known as the **gut microbiome,** which play an essential role in our health. These microorganisms help digest food, synthesize vitamins, regulate immune responses, and protect against harmful pathogens. However, modern lifestyles—rich in processed foods, sugar, and stress—can disrupt this delicate balance, leading to various digestive issues such as bloating, constipation, and even chronic conditions like irritable bowel syndrome (IBS).

A **gut cleanse** is designed to restore balance by removing harmful toxins, reducing inflammation, and fostering an environment where beneficial bacteria can thrive. The benefits of a gut cleanse extend beyond the digestive system, as a healthy gut influences overall wellness, including immune function, mental clarity, energy levels, and even skin health.

Key Benefits of a Gut Cleanse

- **Improved Digestion:** A cleanse helps to remove built-up waste and toxins in the intestines, promoting smoother digestion. It reduces bloating, gas, and constipation while increasing nutrient absorption.
- **Enhanced Gut Flora Balance:** By eliminating harmful substances and introducing prebiotic and probiotic foods, a gut cleanse promotes the growth of beneficial bacteria, which play a critical role in maintaining a balanced gut microbiome.
- **Boosted Energy Levels:** When your gut is healthy and free of toxins, your body can better extract and absorb nutrients from food, providing more energy throughout the day.
- **Reduced Inflammation:** Many digestive issues stem from inflammation within the gut lining. A cleanse helps reduce this inflammation by removing irritating foods and incorporating anti-inflammatory herbs and ingredients.
- **Strengthened Immune System:** A significant portion of the immune system resides in the gut. A well-balanced gut microbiome strengthens the immune response, helping the body fight off infections and reducing the risk of autoimmune conditions.
- **Improved Mental Clarity and Mood:** The **gut-brain axis**—the communication pathway between the gut and the brain—means that gut health directly affects mood and cognitive function. A gut cleanse can alleviate brain fog, improve focus, and reduce anxiety or stress.
- **Clearer Skin:** The gut and skin are closely linked through what's known as the **gut-skin axis.** By reducing inflammation and supporting detoxification, a gut cleanse can lead to clearer, healthier-looking skin.

These benefits demonstrate the significant impact that a healthy gut can have on your overall well-being. Whether you're looking to improve digestion, enhance your energy levels, or strengthen your immune system, a gut cleanse is an essential tool for resetting your body.

Why This Book is Your Go-To Resource

The **15-Day Herbal Gut Reset: Break Free from Failed Detoxes and Reclaim Your Digestive Health** is not just another diet or quick-fix solution—it's a comprehensive, holistic approach to resetting your digestive system and restoring balance to your gut microbiome. This book is your go-to resource for several reasons:

1. Science-Backed Approach

This book is rooted in the latest scientific research on gut health, the microbiome, and the critical role these play in overall wellness. The 15-day cleanse is designed using evidence-based principles that ensure it's safe, effective, and sustainable. The herbal remedies, food recommendations, and lifestyle tips are all based on peer-reviewed studies and real-world results.

2. Focus on Long-Term Results, Not Quick Fixes

Unlike fad diets or detoxes that promise overnight results but deliver little more than temporary water loss, this book is focused on creating long-term changes that support lasting gut health. The 15-day cleanse is designed to kick-start your journey, but it also lays the foundation for lifelong digestive wellness. With practical advice on maintaining a healthy gut post-cleanse, this book ensures you won't just feel better for a few weeks—you'll develop habits that support health for years to come.

3. Holistic Approach to Wellness

This book emphasizes that gut health is not just about what you eat. It integrates the role of mental and emotional well-being into the cleanse, recognizing that stress management, mindfulness, and self-care are crucial to supporting the gut-brain axis. With guidance on mindfulness practices, stress-reduction techniques, and tips for maintaining motivation, this book addresses your health from all angles.

4. Customizable and Flexible

The book is designed to accommodate different lifestyles and dietary preferences. Whether you're vegan, gluten-free, or just looking for ways to integrate more plant-based meals into your diet, the 15-day cleanse offers flexibility. It provides a range of meal plans, recipes, and herbal remedies that can be tailored to your unique needs.

5. Practical and Easy to Follow

This book is packed with actionable steps and easy-to-follow guides, making the cleanse accessible for everyone, whether you're new to gut health or experienced in detoxing. The recipes use readily available ingredients, and the herbal remedies can be easily incorporated into your routine. The included **15-Day Accountability Tracker** ensures that you stay on course, while the **Herbal Remedies Cheat Sheet** provides a quick-reference guide to powerful gut-healing herbs.

How to Use This Book for Maximum Benefit

To make the most out of the **15-Day Herbal Gut Reset,** it's essential to approach the cleanse with the right mindset, follow the steps outlined in the book, and use the tools provided to support your journey. Here's a step-by-step guide on how to use the book for maximum benefit:

1. Read the Introduction and Set Your Goals

Start by reading the Introduction to understand why detoxes often fail and how this cleanse is different. Take a moment to set clear, realistic goals for the cleanse. Do you want to reduce bloating, improve digestion, or boost your energy? Setting specific intentions will keep you motivated and help you measure your progress.

2. Complete the 7-Day Pre-Cleanse Preparation

Before diving into the 15-day cleanse, it's important to prepare your body for the detox. The **7-Day Pre-Cleanse Preparation Guide** outlines steps to gradually reduce your intake of processed foods, sugar, and caffeine while increasing your consumption of whole foods, fiber, and water. Use this phase to stock your kitchen with gut-friendly ingredients, prepare your mindset, and set up a support system.

3. Follow the 15-Day Cleanse Plan

During the cleanse, you'll be following a structured 15-day plan that includes herbal remedies, prebiotic and probiotic foods, and anti-inflammatory meals designed to reset your gut health. Each day, you'll incorporate specific teas, meals, and supplements that nourish your gut, reduce inflammation, and promote detoxification.

Use the **Daily Meal Tracker** and **Hydration & Herbal Tea Tracker** to record your meals, water intake, and herbal teas. These tools will help you stay consistent and ensure that you're meeting the cleanse guidelines. The included recipes are designed to be simple, delicious, and easy to prepare, so you'll have no trouble sticking to the plan.

4. Track Your Symptoms and Non-Scale Victories

As your body detoxifies and your gut heals, you may experience detox symptoms such as fatigue, headaches, or changes in digestion. The **Detox Symptoms Journal** allows you to log these experiences and monitor your progress. Equally important are the **Non-Scale Victories (NSVs)** you'll achieve during the cleanse—such as reduced bloating, clearer skin, or better sleep. Keep track of these positive changes to stay motivated and see how your body responds to the detox.

5. Use the Herbal Remedies Cheat Sheet

Throughout the cleanse, the **Herbal Remedies Cheat Sheet** will be a valuable tool. This quick-reference guide provides information on key digestive herbs, such as ginger, turmeric, and peppermint, and explains how to use them in teas, tinctures, or supplements to support your gut health. Incorporating these herbs into your routine will enhance the benefits of the cleanse and provide long-term digestive support.

6. Stay Active and Practice Self-Care

The book emphasizes that gut health is influenced not only by diet but also by lifestyle factors such as stress management, physical activity, and sleep. Use the **Physical Activity and Movement Log** to track your daily exercise, whether it's a yoga session, a walk, or a strength workout. Additionally, incorporate the **Guided Meditation Series for Gut Health** to reduce stress and support the gut-brain connection.

7. Reflect on Your Progress

At the end of each week, use the **Weekly Reflection** section to review your progress, celebrate your successes, and adjust your plan as needed. Reflecting on your experience will help you stay on track and make any necessary changes to improve your results in the following week.

8. Maintain Long-Term Gut Health Post-Cleanse

After completing the 15-day cleanse, it's important to maintain the progress you've made. The **Post-Cleanse Recipe Book** offers 30 gut-friendly meals that will help you sustain your results and continue supporting your digestive health. Additionally, the book includes long-term strategies, such as incorporating fiber, probiotics, and anti-inflammatory foods into your diet, to ensure you continue reaping the benefits of the cleanse.

A Pathway to Lasting Wellness

The **15-Day Herbal Gut Reset** is more than just a cleanse—it's a guide to lasting wellness. By following the plan, using the tools provided, and staying accountable to your goals, you'll not only reset your gut health but also build the foundation for a healthier, more vibrant life. This book is your trusted resource for reclaiming your digestive health, boosting your energy, and achieving optimal wellness. Whether you're dealing with digestive issues, low energy, or simply looking to enhance your well-being, this book offers a holistic, science-based approach to transform your health from the inside out.

Why Detoxes Fail and How This One Works

Detox programs have become a popular method for individuals looking to reboot their health, lose weight, and restore energy. However, despite the hype surrounding detoxes, many people find themselves cycling through various programs without experiencing the lasting results they were promised. In this introduction, we'll uncover the reasons why so many detoxes fail and explore how this 15-Day Herbal Gut Reset offers a different, scientifically-backed approach to achieve true digestive health and long-lasting vitality.

The Detox Myth: Why So Many Detox Programs Fall Short

Detoxification is often marketed as a quick-fix solution to a myriad of health issues, from weight gain to chronic fatigue. But the truth is, most detox programs oversimplify the complexities of the body's detoxification processes, leaving participants frustrated and without lasting results. Here are some common reasons why detox programs fail:

- **Overly Restrictive Diets:** Many detox programs eliminate entire food groups or require severe calorie restriction, which can lead to nutritional deficiencies, fatigue, and a slow metabolism. Instead of nourishing the body, these programs often do more harm than good.
- **Lack of Support for Gut Health:** Detox programs often focus solely on eliminating toxins but fail to address the health of the digestive system—the body's primary detox organ. Without a healthy gut, toxins cannot be effectively processed and eliminated.
- **Short-Term Focus:** Most detoxes promise dramatic, immediate results, but they neglect the long-term changes needed to maintain health. Participants may lose weight or experience temporary relief, only to find their symptoms return once they resume their normal diet.
- **No Customization:** Detoxes are often marketed as one-size-fits-all, ignoring the unique needs of each person's body and digestive system. Without considering factors like age, activity level, and specific health concerns, these programs are bound to fail some individuals.

The 15-Day Herbal Gut Reset is designed to address these pitfalls by focusing on gut health, utilizing natural remedies that nourish rather than deplete, and offering sustainable, long-term solutions.

The Power of Gut Health: How Your Digestive System Impacts Overall Wellness

The digestive system is much more than a pathway for food; it plays a central role in your overall health and well-being. Known as the "second brain," the gut is home to trillions of bacteria that influence everything from your immune function to your mental clarity and mood. Here's why gut health is critical to detoxification and long-term wellness:

- **Detoxification:** Your liver and kidneys may filter out toxins, but your gut plays a crucial role in eliminating them. If your gut is sluggish or out of balance, toxins can be reabsorbed into your body, leading to inflammation, bloating, and fatigue.
- **Immune Function:** A healthy gut is essential for a strong immune system. In fact, around 70% of your immune cells are located in the gut, making it the first line of defense against harmful pathogens and toxins.
- **Mental Health and Mood:** The gut-brain connection is real. An unhealthy gut can lead to imbalances in neurotransmitters like serotonin, which is responsible for mood regulation. This explains why poor gut health is often linked to anxiety, depression, and brain fog.
- **Nutrient Absorption:** No matter how healthy your diet is, if your gut isn't functioning properly, your body won't absorb the nutrients it needs. Healing the gut allows your body to better assimilate essential vitamins, minerals, and other nutrients.

By focusing on gut health, this 15-day cleanse promotes long-term wellness, energy, and vitality, providing benefits far beyond the typical detox.

Herbal Remedies to the Rescue: What Makes This Cleanse Different and Effective

Unlike typical detoxes that rely on extreme measures like fasting or calorie restriction, the **15-Day Herbal Gut Reset** harnesses the power of natural herbs and whole foods to restore balance to the digestive system. What makes this cleanse different?

- **Herbal Synergy:** The cleanse is built around the use of potent, natural herbs such as ginger, dandelion root, fennel, and milk thistle. These herbs work together to detoxify the liver, soothe inflammation in the gut, and promote healthy digestion. For centuries, herbal remedies have been used to support digestive health, and this program leverages the best of ancient wisdom and modern science.
- **Gut Flora Restoration:** Many detox programs overlook the importance of gut bacteria. This cleanse focuses on replenishing your gut microbiome with prebiotics and probiotics, essential for maintaining a healthy balance of good bacteria. This not only aids digestion but also strengthens the immune system.
- **Whole Food Focus:** Instead of restricting food intake, this cleanse encourages nutrient-dense, anti-inflammatory foods like leafy greens, berries, and fermented products, which support your gut health and provide the fuel your body needs to detox effectively.
- **Sustainable Results:** By avoiding drastic calorie reduction and focusing on nourishing the body, this cleanse sets you up for lasting success. The inclusion of herbal remedies and gut-friendly foods ensures that your digestive system remains balanced and functioning optimally, long after the 15 days are over.

This cleanse is designed for those who have been disappointed by previous detox attempts. It uses a proven, gentle approach that detoxifies while also rebuilding the gut for lasting health improvements.

What to Expect in the Next 15 Days: Setting Realistic Goals and Expectations
Embarking on a cleanse can feel overwhelming, but the 15-Day Herbal Gut Reset is designed to guide you through the process with ease. Here's what you can expect:

- **Gradual Detoxification:** This cleanse does not involve fasting or extreme measures. You'll start by incorporating herbal teas, nutrient-rich smoothies, and prebiotic foods to gently cleanse and restore your gut. Over the first few days, you may notice a reduction in bloating and fatigue as your body starts to detoxify.
- **A Focus on Gut Healing:** As you move into the middle phase of the cleanse, you'll continue to enjoy nourishing meals, fermented foods, and herbal supplements that promote the growth of beneficial bacteria. By the end of the 15 days, your digestive system will feel revitalized and better equipped to process nutrients.
- **Improved Energy and Immunity:** Toward the end of the cleanse, you should experience increased energy, mental clarity, and better immune function. Your body will be detoxifying more efficiently, leaving you feeling lighter, more energetic, and ready to maintain these benefits long-term.

Realistic expectations are key to success. While some benefits may be felt early, such as improved digestion, other results, like enhanced immunity, will become more noticeable as the cleanse progresses.

Before You Begin: Preparing Mentally, Physically, and Nutritionally for the Cleanse
Success in any cleanse depends on adequate preparation. Before starting the 15-Day Herbal Gut Reset, it's important to prepare your body and mind:

- **Mental Preparation:** Set realistic goals for yourself and understand that this is not a quick fix, but a step toward sustainable health. Take time to reflect on your health goals and visualize the long-term benefits you hope to achieve.
- **Physical Preparation:** Begin to phase out processed foods, caffeine, alcohol, and added sugars in the week leading up to the cleanse. This will make the transition easier and help reduce potential detox symptoms like headaches or fatigue.
- **Nutritional Preparation:** Stock your kitchen with whole, fiber-rich foods, herbal supplements, and probiotic-packed items like fermented vegetables or kombucha. Having the right ingredients on hand will make it easier to stick to the program and get the best results.
- **Hydration:** Staying hydrated is crucial during any detox. Start increasing your water intake now to support your body's natural detoxification processes.

By preparing mentally, physically, and nutritionally, you're setting yourself up for success. The 15-Day Herbal Gut Reset is not a sprint, but a journey toward achieving real, lasting digestive health and immune function.

Part 1: The Gut-Immune Connection

Chapter 1:
Understanding Your Gut: The Gateway to Health

In recent years, the scientific community has uncovered a profound truth: our gut is far more than just a place where food is broken down and absorbed. It is a dynamic ecosystem that influences almost every aspect of our health, from digestion and immunity to mental clarity and emotional well-being. The gut is often referred to as the "gateway to health" because its condition reflects and influences the state of our overall wellness. At the heart of this ecosystem is the microbiome—a vast community of bacteria, viruses, fungi, and other microorganisms that live in the digestive tract.

This chapter delves deep into the importance of the gut, how it functions as a critical player in immune health, and how recognizing the signs of gut imbalance is key to reclaiming your health.

The Microbiome Revolution: Why Gut Flora is the Foundation of Health
The term **"microbiome"** refers to the trillions of microorganisms that inhabit your digestive tract. These organisms—comprising bacteria, fungi, viruses, and other microbes—form a diverse community that plays an essential role in maintaining your health. The collective genome of these microbes is known as the **microbiome,** and research into the microbiome has revolutionized our understanding of health.

Here's why the microbiome is so important:

- **Digestion and Nutrient Absorption:** The microbes in your gut break down complex carbohydrates, proteins, and fats, allowing your body to absorb nutrients more efficiently. They also help synthesize essential vitamins, such as B vitamins and vitamin K, which are critical for energy production and blood clotting.
- **Protection Against Pathogens:** A healthy gut microbiome acts as a barrier against harmful bacteria and pathogens. The beneficial bacteria in your gut compete with harmful microbes for space and nutrients, essentially keeping the bad guys at bay. This process helps prevent infections and keeps your digestive system functioning optimally.
- **Metabolic Health:** Your gut flora influences how your body stores fat and regulates glucose metabolism. An imbalanced microbiome can contribute to metabolic disorders such as obesity and type 2 diabetes.
- **Brain Health and Mood Regulation:** The gut and brain are intricately connected through the gut-brain axis. Your gut produces about 90% of the body's serotonin, a neurotransmitter that affects mood, appetite, and sleep. A healthy microbiome can positively influence your mental health, reducing the risk of anxiety, depression, and cognitive decline.
- **Inflammation Control:** The microbiome plays a crucial role in regulating inflammation. Imbalanced gut flora can lead to chronic low-grade inflammation, which is a root cause of many chronic diseases, including heart disease, arthritis, and autoimmune conditions.

The **microbiome revolution** has transformed our understanding of health. No longer can we consider gut health in isolation; instead, it is clear that the health of your microbiome is foundational to the health of your entire body. The delicate balance of this ecosystem is central to your well-being, and maintaining it is one of the most effective ways to prevent disease and promote longevity.

How Gut Health Affects Immunity: Strengthening Your Body's Natural Defense System
Approximately 70% of the immune system is housed in the gut, making the digestive system one of the body's most critical defense systems. The gut and immune system work in tandem to protect the body from harmful invaders like bacteria, viruses, and toxins while maintaining a state of tolerance for beneficial microbes and nutrients.

Here's how gut health and immunity are intertwined:

- **The Gut as the First Line of Defense:** The gut lining acts as a physical barrier that prevents pathogens from entering the bloodstream. Beneficial bacteria in the microbiome help to strengthen this barrier by producing short-chain fatty acids (SCFAs), such as butyrate, which nourish the cells lining the gut. A healthy gut lining ensures that toxins, undigested food particles, and harmful microbes stay within the digestive system, preventing them from triggering an immune response.
- **Modulating Immune Responses:** The microbiome helps to "train" the immune system, teaching it to differentiate between harmful pathogens and harmless substances like food or beneficial bacteria. When the microbiome is balanced, immune cells are less likely to overreact, reducing the risk of autoimmune diseases and allergic reactions. Conversely, an imbalanced gut can lead to immune dysfunction, making the body more prone to chronic inflammation and illness.
- **Producing Antimicrobial Compounds:** Beneficial bacteria in the gut produce compounds that inhibit the growth of harmful bacteria. These natural antibiotics, along with the immune system's production of antibodies, help keep pathogenic microbes in check and prevent infections.
- **Gut-Associated Lymphoid Tissue (GALT):** GALT is a critical component of the immune system that resides in the gut. It contains specialized immune cells that monitor the gut environment for harmful invaders. These immune cells are constantly interacting with the microbiome, responding to changes in the microbial community and triggering appropriate immune responses when necessary.

When the gut microbiome is healthy, the immune system operates efficiently, keeping illness at bay. However, when the microbiome is disrupted, the immune system can become overactive or sluggish, leading to a weakened ability to fight off infections and an increased risk of chronic diseases.

Symptoms of Gut Imbalance: Recognizing the Signs of Poor Gut Health and Immune Dysfunction

A gut that is out of balance can manifest in a variety of ways. Because the gut influences so many bodily systems, the symptoms of an unhealthy microbiome are often far-reaching and not always immediately recognizable as being connected to gut health.

Here are some common signs of **gut imbalance** and immune dysfunction:

- **Digestive Issues:** Symptoms like bloating, gas, constipation, diarrhea, and acid reflux are often the first indicators of an unhealthy gut. These issues arise when the balance of good and bad bacteria is disturbed, leading to poor digestion and nutrient absorption.
- **Chronic Fatigue:** Feeling tired all the time, even after a good night's sleep, can be a sign of gut dysbiosis (imbalance of gut flora). This is because an unhealthy gut can lead to nutrient deficiencies and systemic inflammation, both of which drain your energy.
- **Frequent Infections:** A weakened immune system resulting from poor gut health may lead to frequent colds, flu, and other infections. If you find yourself getting sick often, it may be a sign that your gut isn't functioning optimally.
- **Brain Fog and Mood Swings:** The gut-brain connection means that an imbalanced microbiome can have a direct impact on your mental health. Difficulty concentrating, memory issues, anxiety, depression, and irritability can all be linked to poor gut health.
- **Skin Problems:** Skin conditions like acne, eczema, and rosacea are often signs of inflammation that originate in the gut. When the gut barrier is compromised, toxins can leak into the bloodstream, triggering systemic inflammation that shows up in the skin.
- **Autoimmune Disorders:** Research suggests that poor gut health is a major contributing factor to the development of autoimmune diseases such as rheumatoid arthritis, lupus, and Hashimoto's thyroiditis. When the gut lining is damaged, undigested food particles and toxins can enter the bloodstream, triggering an immune response that may mistakenly target the body's own tissues.
- **Weight Fluctuations:** Unexplained weight gain or loss can be a symptom of gut dysbiosis. An unhealthy gut can interfere with the body's ability to regulate blood sugar, store fat, and manage hunger signals, leading to metabolic imbalances.
- **Food Sensitivities:** An imbalanced gut can increase the likelihood of developing food intolerances, such as sensitivity to gluten, dairy, or sugar. This happens because the immune system becomes overly reactive when the gut is inflamed, mistaking certain foods as threats.

Recognizing these symptoms is the first step toward understanding the need for a gut reset. The good news is that the gut is incredibly resilient, and by restoring balance to the microbiome, you can address these symptoms and support your overall health and immunity.

Your gut is not just a digestive organ—it is the foundation of your overall health. The **microbiome revolution** has shown us that by nourishing the gut and maintaining a healthy balance of gut flora, we can dramatically improve digestion, boost immunity, and enhance mental and emotional well-being. This chapter lays the groundwork for understanding why the gut is central to your health and why focusing on gut balance through a targeted cleanse is the key to unlocking vitality and long-term wellness.

Chapter 2:
How Detoxing Impacts the Immune System

Detoxification is often associated with eliminating toxins for the sake of better digestion or weight loss, but its impact on the immune system is just as significant, if not more so. In fact, a well-executed detox can profoundly influence your immune health by helping your body clear out harmful substances that weaken its defenses. When you detoxify your gut, you're not just cleansing your digestive system; you're giving your immune system the support it needs to function at its best. In this chapter, we'll explore the intricate relationship between toxins, detoxing, and immunity, as well as the herbs that make a gut cleanse particularly effective at boosting immune health.

The Role of Toxins in Immune Suppression: Understanding How Toxins Damage Your System

In our modern world, we are constantly exposed to toxins, whether through the air we breathe, the food we eat, or the products we use. Over time, these toxins accumulate in the body, especially in the gut, and contribute to a wide range of health issues, particularly when it comes to the immune system.

Here's how toxins negatively impact the immune system:

- **Chronic Inflammation:** Toxins such as pesticides, heavy metals, and pollutants trigger the release of inflammatory compounds in the body. This chronic, low-level inflammation weakens the immune system over time, making it less effective at fighting infections and responding to other health threats. Inflammation also leads to damage to tissues and organs, further taxing the immune system.
- **Gut Dysbiosis:** The accumulation of toxins in the gut can disrupt the delicate balance of the gut microbiome, leading to **dysbiosis**—an imbalance between beneficial and harmful bacteria. This imbalance not only affects digestion but also weakens the immune system. Since a significant portion of the immune system resides in the gut, dysbiosis impairs the body's ability to detect and eliminate pathogens effectively.
- **Toxin-Induced Leaky Gut:** Toxins damage the integrity of the gut lining, leading to a condition commonly referred to as **leaky gut syndrome.** This occurs when the tight junctions in the gut lining become loose, allowing toxins, undigested food particles, and harmful microbes to leak into the bloodstream. This leakage triggers an immune response, causing inflammation and overactivation of the immune system, which can eventually lead to autoimmune disorders.
- **Immune Suppression:** Over time, chronic exposure to toxins can directly suppress the activity of immune cells, such as **T-cells** and **B-cells,** which are essential for identifying and neutralizing harmful pathogens. When these cells are compromised, the immune

system struggles to mount an effective response to infections, leaving the body more vulnerable to illness.

- **Toxin Overload:** The liver, kidneys, and gut are responsible for filtering and eliminating toxins, but when these organs become overwhelmed by the volume of toxins, they are unable to function efficiently. This can lead to the reabsorption of toxins into the bloodstream, further burdening the immune system and reducing its ability to fight off disease.

Understanding the role of toxins in immune suppression highlights the importance of detoxification, not just for improving digestion but for strengthening the immune system. By removing toxins from the gut, the immune system is freed from the burden of constantly battling inflammation and can return to its primary role of defending the body against real threats.

Detoxing to Rebalance: How Clearing the Gut Supports Stronger Immunity
Detoxification is not simply about cleansing the digestive system; it's about restoring balance to the body's internal environment, allowing the immune system to function optimally. The gut plays a critical role in this process, as it is both a major site of toxin accumulation and the location of 70% of the immune system.

Here's how detoxing the gut can help rebalance the immune system and strengthen your body's defenses:

- **Restoring Gut Integrity:** A successful detox helps to heal and restore the gut lining, which is crucial for maintaining a healthy immune system. By eliminating the toxins that damage the gut lining and cause **leaky gut,** a detox can reduce the systemic inflammation that often results from these leaks. A stronger gut lining ensures that harmful substances stay within the digestive system and are properly excreted, rather than entering the bloodstream and triggering immune responses.
- **Rebalancing Gut Flora:** A detox, especially one that includes herbal remedies and prebiotic or probiotic-rich foods, can help restore balance to the gut microbiome. By reducing the presence of harmful bacteria and promoting the growth of beneficial bacteria, a detox creates an environment that supports a healthy immune system. A balanced microbiome improves the body's ability to recognize and fight off harmful pathogens, while also preventing overreactions that can lead to autoimmune issues.
- **Supporting Immune Function with Nutrients:** A detox that includes nutrient-rich, anti-inflammatory foods and herbs provides the immune system with the nutrients it needs to function efficiently. For example, **vitamin C, zinc,** and **selenium** are critical for immune cell function, and they are often found in detox-friendly foods like leafy greens, citrus fruits, and nuts. By replenishing these essential nutrients, a detox helps to nourish the immune system.

- **Reducing Toxin-Induced Inflammation:** By eliminating the toxins that contribute to chronic inflammation, a detox gives the immune system a chance to reset. With lower levels of inflammation, immune cells can focus on identifying and neutralizing real threats, such as viruses and bacteria, rather than being overactive in response to toxins and damaged tissues.
- **Enhancing Lymphatic Function:** The lymphatic system, which is closely tied to the immune system, plays a vital role in removing toxins from the body. A gut detox can improve lymphatic drainage by reducing the load of toxins the body has to process. This, in turn, improves immune function, as the lymphatic system is responsible for transporting immune cells to areas where they are needed most.

Detoxing the gut is one of the most effective ways to strengthen the immune system. By clearing out harmful substances, restoring balance to the microbiome, and reducing inflammation, detoxification creates an environment where the immune system can thrive. This rebalance is especially important for individuals who have been exposed to high levels of environmental toxins or have experienced frequent illnesses, as it provides a pathway to restoring optimal immune function.

Herbs for Immunity: The Key Ingredients in Your Cleanse That Boost Immune Response
Herbal remedies have been used for centuries to support both detoxification and immunity. In the **15-Day Herbal Gut Reset,** several powerful herbs are included to boost immune function while cleansing the gut. These herbs not only help eliminate toxins but also provide immune-boosting benefits that support long-term health.

Here are some of the key herbs included in your cleanse and how they boost immunity:

- **Ginger:** Ginger is a powerful anti-inflammatory herb that helps soothe the digestive system while supporting immune function. It contains compounds called **gingerols** and **shogaols** that have been shown to enhance immune response by reducing inflammation and promoting healthy circulation. Ginger also supports detoxification by stimulating digestion and promoting the elimination of toxins through the bowels.
- **Turmeric:** Known for its anti-inflammatory and antioxidant properties, turmeric contains **curcumin,** a compound that supports the immune system by reducing chronic inflammation and enhancing the activity of immune cells. Turmeric also helps protect the gut lining and reduces the risk of leaky gut, which can trigger immune dysfunction.
- **Dandelion Root:** Dandelion root is a natural detoxifier that supports liver function, one of the body's main organs of detoxification. By promoting bile production and aiding digestion, dandelion root helps the body eliminate toxins more efficiently. It also has immune-boosting properties due to its high antioxidant content, which protects immune cells from oxidative stress.

- **Echinacea:** Echinacea is a well-known immune stimulant that has been shown to increase the activity of white blood cells, the body's first line of defense against infections. Echinacea also has antiviral and anti-inflammatory properties, making it an excellent herb for strengthening the immune system during detoxification.
- **Garlic:** Garlic contains **allicin,** a compound that has potent antimicrobial properties. It helps boost immune function by stimulating the production of **T-cells** and enhancing the ability of immune cells to fight infections. Garlic also supports detoxification by promoting healthy digestion and reducing harmful bacteria in the gut.
- **Milk Thistle:** Milk thistle is a liver-supporting herb that helps the body process and eliminate toxins. It contains **silymarin,** a compound that protects liver cells from damage and supports the regeneration of new liver cells. By supporting liver function, milk thistle ensures that the body can efficiently remove toxins, reducing the burden on the immune system.
- **Astragalus:** Astragalus is an adaptogen that helps the body cope with stress while also boosting immune function. It enhances the production of white blood cells and has been shown to improve the body's ability to fight off viral infections. Astragalus also has anti-inflammatory properties that support gut health and immune function.

Including these herbs in your detox not only supports the elimination of toxins but also strengthens your immune system. By reducing inflammation, protecting immune cells, and promoting a balanced microbiome, these herbs help create an environment where your immune system can function at its best.

 In this chapter, we've explored the critical role toxins play in suppressing immune function and how detoxing the gut can help restore balance and strengthen immunity. By removing harmful substances, healing the gut lining, and supporting the immune system with powerful herbs, a targeted detox can provide long-lasting benefits for both digestive and immune health. As you embark on your **15-Day Herbal Gut Reset,** you'll be supporting your immune system in ways that go beyond just improving digestion—you'll be building a stronger, more resilient body that can better defend itself against illness and disease.

Part 2: Why Previous Detoxes Didn't Work (And How This One Will)

Chapter 3:
Common Pitfalls in Traditional Detox Programs

Detox programs are often marketed as miracle solutions, promising rapid results with little effort. However, these quick-fix approaches often fall short of delivering long-lasting benefits and, in many cases, can even harm your body. In this chapter, we will explore the common pitfalls that make traditional detox programs ineffective. We will also debunk some of the myths surrounding detoxing and explain why incorporating herbal remedies is the missing link that can transform a typical cleanse into a sustainable and health-promoting regimen.

Why Quick-Fix Detoxes Fail: The Danger of Overly Restrictive Diets

One of the most common features of traditional detox programs is the promise of rapid results in a very short amount of time, often with minimal effort. These programs typically involve **overly restrictive diets** that may exclude entire food groups, significantly limit caloric intake, or rely on only liquid consumption. While these methods can produce short-term changes, they often fail to deliver lasting results and can come with significant downsides.

Here's why quick-fix detoxes fall short:

- **Starvation Mode:** Many detox programs require participants to drastically reduce their caloric intake, sometimes to levels that can trigger the body's **starvation response.** When the body is deprived of calories, it slows down the metabolism in an effort to conserve energy. This can lead to initial weight loss, but as soon as the individual resumes normal eating patterns, the weight often returns—sometimes even more than before. This yo-yo effect leaves many feeling disillusioned and frustrated.
- **Nutrient Deficiencies:** Overly restrictive detoxes often eliminate critical nutrients that your body needs to function properly. Programs that require participants to consume only juice, for example, lack the essential proteins, fats, and fibers that are necessary for healthy metabolism, muscle maintenance, and digestive health. Long-term nutrient deficiencies can weaken the immune system, lead to muscle loss, and impair overall health.
- **Muscle Breakdown:** When the body is deprived of protein and other essential nutrients, it begins to break down muscle tissue for energy. This can cause a significant loss of muscle mass, which is not only detrimental to physical strength and endurance but also to metabolism. Muscle is metabolically active tissue, meaning it burns more calories than fat, even at rest. Losing muscle can make it harder to maintain a healthy weight over time.
- **Rebound Weight Gain:** The problem with rapid weight loss programs is that they don't address the root causes of weight gain. By focusing solely on caloric restriction or food elimination, quick-fix detoxes fail to change unhealthy eating habits or support the body's natural detoxification pathways. When the detox ends and normal eating resumes, the body is more likely to regain weight because the underlying issues have not been addressed. The weight gained after detoxing is often more stubborn and harder to lose.

- **Emotional and Mental Stress:** Severe caloric restriction or highly restrictive food lists can lead to feelings of deprivation, irritability, and stress. In many cases, participants feel compelled to quit the detox early, feeling that the program is too difficult to maintain. This can leave them feeling like they've failed, contributing to a cycle of guilt and unhealthy relationship with food.

The bottom line is that **overly restrictive diets** in detox programs are not sustainable. They may produce immediate results, but they do not set the stage for long-term health and wellness. Instead of focusing on rapid weight loss or extreme measures, a successful detox must support the body's natural processes and provide nourishment, rather than deprivation.

Debunking Detox Myths: Clearing Up the Misinformation About Cleansing
The popularity of detox programs has led to a wide range of myths and misconceptions about how detoxification works and what it can achieve. Many of these myths are perpetuated by marketing claims that prioritize sales over scientific accuracy. Let's clear up some of the most common myths about detoxing:

1. Myth: Detoxing Can Be Done in a Day or Two

- **Fact:** The idea that you can fully detox your body in just a day or two is a major misconception. Detoxification is a complex, ongoing process that your body performs naturally every day. While certain practices can support and enhance this process, true detoxification, particularly in the gut and liver, takes time. A more realistic and effective approach is to engage in a detox plan that lasts long enough to address accumulated toxins and restore balance to the body, typically over a period of 7-15 days.

2. Myth: Detoxing Is Only About Weight Loss

- **Fact:** While weight loss can be a byproduct of detoxing, it should never be the primary goal. A detox is about removing toxins from the body, improving digestion, and supporting overall health. Focusing solely on weight loss can lead to misguided approaches, such as extreme calorie cutting, which can be counterproductive. A successful detox improves digestive health, supports immune function, enhances energy levels, and promotes mental clarity—weight loss, if needed, should be a secondary benefit, not the primary goal.

3. Myth: Juice Cleanses Are the Best Way to Detox

- **Fact:** Juice cleanses are often marketed as a quick and effective way to detox, but they come with significant downsides. While they may provide a temporary boost in vitamins and hydration, juice cleanses often lack the fiber, protein, and healthy fats needed to maintain energy levels, support gut health, and build muscle. Without these essential nutrients, participants may feel fatigued, weak, and unable to sustain the cleanse. Additionally, juice cleanses can cause blood sugar spikes and crashes, leading to mood swings and cravings.

4. Myth: Detox Supplements Alone Can Fix Everything

- **Fact:** There's no magic pill or supplement that can single-handedly detoxify the body. While certain supplements, such as herbal extracts or probiotics, can support the body's natural detox processes, they must be part of a broader approach that includes proper nutrition, hydration, and lifestyle changes. Supplements alone are not enough to effectively cleanse the body or restore gut health.

5. Myth: Detoxing Is Unnecessary Because the Body Naturally Cleanses Itself

- **Fact:** While it is true that the body has its own detoxification systems (primarily through the liver, kidneys, skin, and lungs), modern life exposes us to an unprecedented amount of toxins from processed foods, environmental pollutants, and chemicals in personal care products. These toxins can overwhelm the body's natural detox processes, leading to the accumulation of harmful substances in the body. Supporting the body with periodic detoxes can help reduce this burden and enhance the function of the liver, gut, and other detox organs.

By debunking these myths, it becomes clear that detoxing is not about quick fixes or drastic measures. Instead, it's about supporting the body's natural processes with the right tools, timing, and nutrition. This is where herbal remedies come into play as the missing link that elevates detoxing from a short-term trend to a sustainable health practice.

The Missing Link: Why Herbal Remedies Are the Secret Weapon in a Successful Cleanse
Herbal remedies have been used for thousands of years across various cultures to support digestion, cleanse the body, and enhance overall health. In the modern era, they remain a powerful and effective tool in detox programs, offering benefits that many traditional detoxes overlook.

Here's why **herbal remedies** are the missing link in most detox programs and why they make a significant difference in a successful cleanse:

- **Supporting the Liver:** The liver is the body's primary detox organ, responsible for filtering toxins from the blood and breaking them down so they can be eliminated. Herbal remedies such as **milk thistle** and **dandelion root** are known to support liver function by boosting its ability to detoxify and regenerate. These herbs provide antioxidants that protect liver cells from damage and enhance the liver's capacity to process toxins more efficiently.
- **Promoting Gut Health:** Many traditional detox programs focus solely on the liver and kidneys but neglect the gut, where a significant portion of detoxification takes place. Herbs like **slippery elm, marshmallow root,** and **licorice root** are excellent for soothing inflammation in the gut, repairing the gut lining, and improving the elimination of waste. By promoting gut health, these herbs also help reduce bloating, improve digestion, and ensure that toxins are efficiently excreted from the body.

- **Balancing the Microbiome:** A healthy microbiome is essential for a successful detox, as beneficial bacteria help metabolize toxins and prevent harmful bacteria from proliferating. **Probiotic-rich herbs** like **astragalus** and **burdock root** help nourish the gut microbiome, supporting the growth of beneficial bacteria and enhancing the body's ability to process and eliminate toxins.
- **Reducing Inflammation:** Inflammation is often a byproduct of toxin buildup, and chronic inflammation can lead to a weakened immune system, fatigue, and digestive issues. Herbs like **turmeric, ginger,** and **boswellia** have potent anti-inflammatory properties that help reduce inflammation throughout the body. By calming inflammation, these herbs support the immune system, reduce pain, and enhance the detox process.
- **Enhancing Elimination:** Effective detoxification depends on the body's ability to eliminate toxins through the bowels, urine, and sweat. Herbs like **senna, cascara sagrada,** and **aloe vera** are natural laxatives that gently stimulate bowel movements, ensuring that waste is promptly removed from the body. Diuretic herbs like **parsley** and **nettle** increase urine production, supporting kidney function and helping to flush out water-soluble toxins.
- **Boosting Immunity:** A successful detox isn't just about removing toxins; it's also about fortifying the body's defenses so it can better handle future exposures to toxins. Herbs like **echinacea, garlic,** and **elderberry** boost immune function, helping the body fight off infections and recover more quickly from illness. These herbs are rich in antioxidants and compounds that stimulate the production of white blood cells, which are essential for a robust immune response.

Herbal remedies provide a holistic approach to detoxification that supports the body's natural processes without the harsh side effects of extreme diets or synthetic supplements. By incorporating these time-tested herbs into a cleanse, participants can experience deeper, more sustainable results, including improved digestion, enhanced immunity, and long-term health benefits.

Traditional detox programs often fall short because they rely on restrictive diets, unrealistic promises, and a focus on short-term results. However, by understanding the pitfalls of quick-fix detoxes, debunking common detox myths, and integrating powerful herbal remedies, you can create a detox that supports your body's natural cleansing processes and promotes long-lasting health. Herbal remedies are the **missing link** that elevate detox programs, helping you achieve better digestion, stronger immunity, and sustainable wellness. As you move forward in the **15-Day Herbal Gut Reset,** you'll discover how these natural tools can transform your approach to detoxing and provide real, lasting results.

Chapter 4:
The Science Behind a Successful Herbal Detox

In the world of detoxing, there's a lot of misinformation and quick-fix solutions that overlook the complexity of the body's detoxification processes. A successful detox goes beyond simply eliminating toxins; it involves nourishing the body, restoring balance, and supporting long-term health, particularly through the gut. The use of herbal remedies in detoxing is a time-tested practice rooted in ancient medicine and increasingly backed by modern science. This chapter delves into the science behind how herbal detox works, focusing on how herbs can synergize to cleanse the body, how prebiotics and probiotics restore gut flora, and how a healthy gut directly influences immune function.

Herbal Synergy: How Herbs Work Together to Cleanse and Heal the Gut

Herbal remedies are at the core of many detox programs, but what sets them apart in a successful herbal detox is their ability to work in **synergy.** Synergy occurs when the combined effect of two or more herbs is greater than the sum of their individual effects. This concept is especially important in detoxing, where multiple organs and systems must work together to remove toxins and restore health.

Here's how **herbal synergy** works in a gut-focused detox:

Liver and Digestive Support: The liver plays a central role in detoxification, filtering toxins from the bloodstream and metabolizing them for elimination. Herbs like **milk thistle** and **dandelion root** are commonly used to support liver function. Milk thistle contains a compound called **silymarin,** which has been shown to protect liver cells from damage and promote regeneration. Dandelion root, meanwhile, stimulates bile production, which aids in digestion and helps the liver more efficiently process and eliminate toxins. When used together, these herbs enhance liver detoxification while also supporting digestive health.

Gut Soothing and Healing: Many toxins, particularly those found in processed foods, alcohol, and medications, can irritate the gut lining, leading to conditions like **leaky gut syndrome.** Herbs like **slippery elm, marshmallow root,** and **licorice root** work together to soothe and heal the digestive tract. Slippery elm and marshmallow root contain mucilage, a gel-like substance that coats the digestive tract, reducing inflammation and promoting healing of the gut lining. Licorice root helps reduce inflammation while also balancing cortisol levels, which can become elevated due to chronic stress and poor diet. These herbs, when combined, provide comprehensive support for healing the gut, reducing inflammation, and restoring digestive integrity.

Cleansing and Elimination: Effective detoxification requires that toxins are not only processed but also eliminated from the body through the bowels and urine. **Senna, cascara sagrada,** and **aloe vera** are natural laxatives that gently stimulate bowel movements, ensuring that waste is properly expelled. Meanwhile, **nettle** and **parsley** are mild diuretics that help the kidneys flush out water-soluble toxins through urine. By combining these herbs, the detox ensures that toxins are not reabsorbed into the body but are efficiently eliminated, reducing the risk of toxin buildup.

Anti-Inflammatory and Antioxidant Properties: Many herbs used in detox programs are rich in anti-inflammatory compounds and antioxidants. **Turmeric,** for example, contains **curcumin,** a powerful anti-inflammatory agent that helps reduce inflammation in the gut and throughout the body. **Ginger** also has potent anti-inflammatory properties and supports digestion by stimulating gastric motility. **Garlic** provides antioxidant protection by neutralizing free radicals, which can damage cells and lead to chronic inflammation. When used in synergy, these herbs create a powerful anti-inflammatory and antioxidant effect, which helps the body detoxify more efficiently and reduces the harmful effects of toxin exposure.

Herbal synergy is essential to a successful detox because it allows different herbs to target multiple aspects of the detoxification process—supporting the liver, healing the gut, promoting elimination, and reducing inflammation—all at the same time. By leveraging the unique properties of each herb, a well-designed herbal detox can provide comprehensive support for the body, leading to lasting results.

Gut Flora Restoration: Using Prebiotics and Probiotics to Reset the Microbiome
A successful detox doesn't just remove toxins from the body; it also **restores balance to the gut microbiome,** which plays a crucial role in digestion, immune function, and overall health. The microbiome is the community of trillions of bacteria, viruses, and fungi that live in the gut, and its health is closely tied to the health of the entire body.

Toxins, poor diet, stress, and antibiotics can disrupt the microbiome, leading to **dysbiosis**—an imbalance between beneficial and harmful bacteria in the gut. This imbalance can result in a variety of health problems, including bloating, indigestion, weakened immunity, and even mental health issues like anxiety and depression.

The **15-Day Herbal Gut Reset** focuses on restoring the microbiome through the use of **prebiotics** and **probiotics:**

- **Prebiotics: Feeding the Good Bacteria:** Prebiotics are non-digestible fibers that serve as food for beneficial gut bacteria. By consuming prebiotics, you promote the growth of good bacteria in the gut, helping to restore balance to the microbiome. Foods like **chicory root, asparagus, garlic, onions,** and **bananas** are rich in prebiotics and can be easily incorporated into a detox plan. Herbal sources of prebiotics, such as **burdock root** and **dandelion root,** are also effective at nourishing the microbiome. By feeding the good bacteria, prebiotics help strengthen the gut's natural defenses and improve digestion.
- **Probiotics: Replenishing Beneficial Bacteria:** Probiotics are live bacteria that help restore the balance of the microbiome. Consuming probiotic-rich foods like **yogurt, kefir,**

sauerkraut, kimchi, and **miso** during a detox can replenish the good bacteria that have been depleted by poor diet, stress, or medication use. In addition to fermented foods, herbal supplements that contain probiotics, such as **lactobacillus** and **bifidobacterium,** can help speed up the restoration process. Probiotics improve digestion, enhance immune function, and reduce inflammation in the gut, making them a critical component of any detox program.

- **The Role of Synbiotics:** The combination of prebiotics and probiotics is known as **synbiotics,** and together, they work synergistically to restore the microbiome. Prebiotics provide the necessary fuel for probiotics to thrive, creating a healthy environment for beneficial bacteria to multiply. By incorporating both into your detox program, you can reset the microbiome more effectively, improving gut health and supporting the detoxification process.

Restoring gut flora through the use of prebiotics and probiotics not only improves digestion and nutrient absorption but also enhances immune function, reduces inflammation, and supports mental health. A healthy microbiome is essential for long-term wellness, and by focusing on microbiome restoration during a detox, you can set the stage for lasting health benefits.

The Immune System Link: Rebuilding Immunity Through the Gut
The gut is often referred to as the "second brain" because of its profound influence on the body, particularly on the immune system. In fact, approximately 70% of the immune system resides in the gut, where it interacts with the microbiome to protect the body from harmful pathogens while maintaining tolerance to beneficial bacteria and harmless substances.

Here's how a healthy gut supports a robust immune system, and how detoxing the gut can help rebuild immunity:

- **The Gut-Immune Axis:** The gut and immune system are in constant communication through a network of immune cells located in the **gut-associated lymphoid tissue (GALT).** This system monitors the contents of the gut and determines whether an immune response is needed. A healthy microbiome supports the immune system by promoting the production of regulatory **T-cells,** which help modulate immune responses and prevent the immune system from overreacting to harmless substances (as occurs in autoimmune diseases and allergies).
- **Reducing Inflammation:** Chronic inflammation is a major contributor to immune dysfunction, and much of this inflammation originates in the gut. Toxins, poor diet, and dysbiosis can all trigger inflammation, leading to a weakened immune system. By detoxing the gut and restoring balance to the microbiome, you can reduce systemic inflammation and support a healthy immune response. Herbs like **turmeric, ginger,** and **boswellia** are powerful anti-inflammatory agents that help calm the immune system and reduce the inflammatory load on the body.

- **Rebuilding Gut Barrier Function:** The gut lining acts as a barrier that prevents harmful substances from entering the bloodstream. When this barrier is compromised (as in **leaky gut syndrome),** toxins and undigested food particles can pass through, triggering an immune response. This can lead to chronic inflammation, autoimmunity, and other immune-related issues. A successful detox helps to rebuild the gut lining through the use of healing herbs like **slippery elm** and **licorice root,** which soothe and repair the gut barrier. A healthy gut lining ensures that only beneficial nutrients are absorbed, while harmful substances are eliminated, reducing the burden on the immune system.

- **Strengthening Immune Defense:** Certain herbs used in detox programs, such as **echinacea, garlic,** and **astragalus,** are known for their immune-boosting properties. These herbs help stimulate the production of **white blood cells** (the body's primary defense against infection) and enhance the activity of **macrophages,** which are responsible for engulfing and destroying pathogens. By incorporating immune-supporting herbs into a detox, you can strengthen your body's defenses and improve its ability to fend off illness.

- **Enhancing Immune Tolerance:** A balanced microbiome is essential for maintaining **immune tolerance,** the ability of the immune system to distinguish between harmful pathogens and harmless substances like food and beneficial bacteria. Dysbiosis and toxin overload can disrupt this balance, leading to autoimmune diseases, food sensitivities, and allergies. A gut detox that focuses on restoring the microbiome can help the immune system regain its ability to tolerate harmless substances while mounting an appropriate defense against real threats.

Rebuilding immunity through the gut is one of the most important benefits of a successful detox. By reducing inflammation, restoring the gut barrier, and supporting immune cell function, detoxing the gut provides a foundation for long-term immune health. As you progress through the **15-Day Herbal Gut Reset,** your immune system will become more resilient, better equipped to handle the challenges of modern life, and less prone to infections, allergies, and autoimmune issues.

The science behind a successful herbal detox lies in understanding how herbs work together to cleanse and heal the gut, how prebiotics and probiotics restore the microbiome, and how a healthy gut supports a strong immune system. By focusing on these key elements, the **15-Day Herbal Gut Reset** goes beyond traditional detox programs, offering a holistic approach that promotes not only detoxification but also long-term health and resilience. As you continue with the cleanse, you'll experience the transformative power of herbal synergy, microbiome restoration, and immune system support—setting the stage for lasting wellness.

Part 3: The 15-Day Herbal Gut Cleanse Plan

Chapter 5:
Preparing for Your Cleanse

Embarking on a cleanse, especially one as comprehensive as the **15-Day Herbal Gut Reset,** requires preparation. Detoxing is a transformative journey, and like any journey, being well-prepared is key to success. While the cleanse itself is designed to gently support your body through a process of healing and detoxification, preparing your mind, body, and kitchen beforehand will ensure that you get the most out of the experience. This chapter covers everything you need to know before starting your cleanse, from dietary changes and essential herbs to stocking your kitchen with the right ingredients and setting realistic goals for the journey ahead.

Pre-Cleanse Preparation: Diet Changes, Hydration, and Mental Readiness

Before diving into your cleanse, it's essential to prepare your body and mind for the process. A cleanse can be physically demanding, especially in the early stages when your body is adjusting to new habits and detoxifying accumulated toxins. However, with proper pre-cleanse preparation, you can ease this transition and set yourself up for a smoother, more effective detox experience.

Diet Changes

In the week leading up to your cleanse, it's a good idea to begin making gradual dietary changes that align with the principles of the detox. This will help your body adjust and reduce the likelihood of experiencing detox symptoms like headaches, fatigue, or cravings in the first few days.

- **Eliminate Processed Foods:** Processed foods, including those high in added sugars, refined grains, and artificial additives, are some of the biggest contributors to toxin accumulation. Begin phasing out processed snacks, fast food, sugary drinks, and packaged foods to reduce the toxic load on your body before the cleanse even begins.
- **Cut Back on Caffeine and Alcohol:** Both caffeine and alcohol are taxing on the liver, the body's primary detoxification organ. In the week leading up to your cleanse, gradually reduce your intake of coffee, alcohol, and other stimulants. This will help minimize withdrawal symptoms such as headaches and irritability once you start the cleanse.
- **Increase Whole Foods:** Focus on eating whole, nutrient-dense foods like fruits, vegetables, whole grains, lean proteins, and healthy fats. These foods are rich in the vitamins, minerals, and antioxidants your body needs to support detoxification and maintain energy during the cleanse. Leafy greens, cruciferous vegetables, berries, nuts, seeds, and avocados are all great choices.
- **Transition to Plant-Based:** If your cleanse emphasizes a plant-based approach, begin incorporating more plant-based meals into your daily diet. This will help your digestive system adjust to higher fiber intake and reduce the shock to your system when you fully adopt a plant-based cleanse.

Hydration

Proper hydration is critical during detoxification, as water helps flush toxins out of the body through the kidneys, liver, and skin. In the days leading up to your cleanse, increase your water intake to at least 8-10 glasses per day. You can also incorporate **herbal teas** and **coconut water** to stay hydrated and replenish electrolytes. Hydration also supports digestion, reduces bloating, and helps prevent fatigue during the cleanse.

Some tips for hydration during the pre-cleanse phase include:

- **Start the Day with Water:** Drink a large glass of water with a slice of lemon first thing in the morning to kickstart digestion and help flush out toxins.
- **Carry a Water Bottle:** Keeping a water bottle with you throughout the day will remind you to sip water consistently, ensuring you stay hydrated.
- **Incorporate Herbal Teas:** Teas like **peppermint, ginger,** and **dandelion root** can soothe digestion and gently support detoxification in the days leading up to the cleanse.

Mental Readiness

Cleansing is not just a physical process; it also requires mental and emotional preparation. As you prepare for your cleanse, take time to set intentions and focus on your goals. Consider keeping a journal where you can document your reasons for cleansing, your expectations, and any concerns you may have. This can help you stay motivated and grounded during the cleanse.

- **Visualize Success:** Spend a few minutes each day visualizing how you'll feel once the cleanse is complete—lighter, more energized, and with improved digestion and mental clarity. This positive visualization can boost your resolve and help you stay committed.
- **Acknowledge Challenges:** Recognize that there may be challenges along the way, whether it's resisting cravings, feeling fatigued, or experiencing detox symptoms. By acknowledging these potential hurdles in advance, you'll be better equipped to handle them when they arise.

Herbal Essentials: The Key Herbs You'll Need for a Successful Cleanse
Herbs are at the heart of the **15-Day Herbal Gut Reset,** providing powerful detoxifying and healing properties that enhance your body's ability to cleanse. Each herb in the cleanse has a specific role in supporting digestion, detoxification, and immune function.

Here are the **key herbs** you'll need for a successful cleanse, along with their benefits:

Milk Thistle

Milk thistle is one of the most well-known herbs for liver support. It contains a compound called **silymarin,** which helps protect liver cells from damage, promotes regeneration of liver tissue, and enhances the liver's ability to detoxify toxins. As the liver is the body's primary detox organ, milk thistle plays a vital role in ensuring that toxins are efficiently processed and eliminated.

Dandelion Root

Dandelion root is a powerful digestive tonic and liver detoxifier. It stimulates bile production, which aids in fat digestion and helps the liver remove waste more efficiently. Dandelion root is also a diuretic, meaning it helps the kidneys eliminate excess water and toxins from the body through urine.

Slippery Elm

Slippery elm is a soothing herb that helps heal the lining of the digestive tract. It contains mucilage, a gel-like substance that coats the stomach and intestines, reducing inflammation and promoting healing of the gut lining. This is particularly important for those dealing with **leaky gut syndrome** or other digestive issues.

Turmeric

Turmeric is a potent anti-inflammatory herb that supports both digestion and detoxification. Its active compound, **curcumin,** helps reduce inflammation in the gut and liver, making it easier for the body to eliminate toxins. Turmeric also has antioxidant properties that protect cells from free radical damage.

Ginger

Ginger is a warming herb that stimulates digestion and helps relieve nausea, bloating, and gas. It increases gastric motility, ensuring that food moves smoothly through the digestive system, and supports the body's natural detoxification processes by enhancing circulation and promoting sweating.

Peppermint

Peppermint is a soothing herb for the digestive system, helping to reduce bloating, indigestion, and gas. It also has mild antimicrobial properties, which can help balance the gut microbiome by inhibiting the growth of harmful bacteria.

Senna

Senna is a natural laxative that helps stimulate bowel movements, ensuring that toxins and waste are efficiently eliminated from the body. While it should be used sparingly, senna is an effective herb for relieving constipation and supporting detoxification through the bowels.

By incorporating these herbs into your cleanse, you'll enhance your body's ability to detoxify while also soothing and healing the gut. These herbs can be consumed in the form of **teas, tinctures, or supplements,** depending on your preference and the specific cleanse protocol you're following.

Kitchen Staples: Stocking Up on Fiber-Rich Foods, Fermented Products, and Herbal Supplements

A successful cleanse relies on more than just herbs—you'll also need to nourish your body with whole, nutrient-dense foods that support detoxification and promote gut health. Stocking your kitchen with the right ingredients will make it easier to stick to the cleanse and maximize its benefits.

Here's a list of **kitchen staples** you'll need for your cleanse:

Fiber-Rich Foods

Fiber is essential for supporting digestion and promoting the elimination of waste. It helps regulate bowel movements, prevents constipation, and binds to toxins in the gut so they can be excreted from the body.

- **Leafy Greens** (spinach, kale, arugula)
- **Cruciferous Vegetables** (broccoli, cauliflower, Brussels sprouts)
- **Whole Grains** (quinoa, brown rice, oats)
- **Legumes** (lentils, chickpeas, black beans)
- **Seeds** (chia seeds, flaxseeds, pumpkin seeds)

Fermented Products

Fermented foods are rich in probiotics, which help restore balance to the gut microbiome. Incorporating fermented foods into your cleanse will support digestion, boost immune function, and reduce inflammation.

- **Sauerkraut**
- **Kimchi**
- **Kefir**
- **Miso**
- **Tempeh**

Herbal Supplements

In addition to consuming herbs through teas and tinctures, you may want to supplement with specific herbal extracts that support detoxification and gut health. Look for high-quality supplements that contain the key herbs listed earlier in this chapter.

- **Milk Thistle Extract**
- **Dandelion Root Capsules**
- **Turmeric with Black Pepper**
- **Probiotic Supplements** (with multiple strains of beneficial bacteria)

Having these ingredients on hand will ensure that you're well-equipped to follow the cleanse and nourish your body with the nutrients it needs for successful detoxification.

Setting Realistic Goals: What You Should Expect Each Week of the Cleanse

One of the most important aspects of a successful cleanse is setting realistic goals. While it's tempting to expect immediate results, detoxing is a gradual process, and it's important to give your body time to adjust. By setting expectations for each week of the cleanse, you can stay motivated and focused on the long-term benefits.

Week 1: Gentle Detox and Adjustment

During the first week, your body will begin the detox process by gradually eliminating toxins from the liver, kidneys, and digestive system. You may experience some mild detox symptoms, such as headaches, fatigue, or irritability, as your body adjusts to the cleanse.

- **Focus:** Supporting liver function and enhancing digestion.
- **Expected Results:** Increased bowel movements, reduced bloating, and a slight increase in energy by the end of the week.

Week 2: Deep Cleansing and Gut Healing

In the second week, your body will enter a deeper phase of detoxification, focusing on healing the gut and restoring balance to the microbiome. You should begin to feel more energized and notice improvements in digestion and mental clarity.

- **Focus:** Healing the gut lining, reducing inflammation, and restoring gut flora.
- **Expected Results:** Improved digestion, less bloating, increased energy, and mental clarity.

Week 3: Revitalization and Rebuilding

By the third week, your body will be in full detox mode, and you should feel lighter, more energized, and less bloated. Your gut will be healing, and your immune system will be stronger.

- **Focus:** Strengthening the immune system and maintaining a healthy gut microbiome.
- **Expected Results:** Increased vitality, better digestion, clearer skin, and improved immunity.

Setting these weekly goals will help you track your progress and stay motivated throughout the cleanse. Remember that everyone's body is different, so listen to your body and adjust as needed.

Proper preparation is essential for a successful cleanse. By making small dietary changes, staying hydrated, gathering the right herbs, and stocking your kitchen with nutrient-dense foods, you're setting the stage for a transformative experience. As you embark on the **15-Day Herbal Gut Reset,** remember to set realistic goals and be patient with your body as it detoxifies and heals. The benefits of this cleanse go beyond temporary results—it's about creating a foundation for long-term health and wellness.

Chapter 6:
Days 1-5: Resetting Your Digestive System

The first five days of the **15-Day Herbal Gut Reset** are crucial for laying the foundation of your cleanse. This is the period when your body starts adjusting to the new diet, herbs, and lifestyle changes. These early days are all about resetting your digestive system, reducing the toxic load, and preparing your gut for the deeper healing that will follow in the later stages of the cleanse.

In this chapter, we'll explore how to ease into the cleanse, establish daily detox rituals that nourish and cleanse, manage common detox symptoms, and incorporate fiber and fermented foods to restore balance to your gut flora.

Getting Started: How to Ease Into the Cleanse Without Shock to Your System

The initial days of any detox can feel like a shock to the system, particularly if your body is used to processed foods, caffeine, sugar, or alcohol. To avoid overwhelming your body, it's essential to ease into the cleanse gently, allowing your digestive system to adjust gradually to the new routines and dietary changes.

Here's how to ease into the cleanse and ensure a smooth start:

1. Start Slow with Dietary Changes

If you haven't already made pre-cleanse adjustments, begin by gradually eliminating processed foods, sugar, caffeine, and alcohol. Rather than cutting them out all at once, phase them out over the first couple of days to minimize withdrawal symptoms. This will allow your body to adjust without triggering severe cravings or detox reactions.

- **Day 1-2:** Focus on eating whole foods such as fruits, vegetables, whole grains, and lean proteins while cutting back on processed snacks and sugary foods.
- **Day 3-5:** Transition into more plant-based meals, adding in fiber-rich foods, probiotics, and herbal teas.

2. Prioritize Hydration

Proper hydration is critical during the first five days. Your body will start flushing out toxins, and staying hydrated helps support kidney function and prevents headaches, fatigue, and constipation, which can arise during detox.

- Drink at least 8-10 glasses of water each day, and add lemon or apple cider vinegar to your water to enhance detoxification.
- **Herbal teas** like peppermint, dandelion root, and ginger are excellent for hydration and have additional detoxifying properties.

3. Begin Your Herbal Detox Rituals Early

It's important to start incorporating herbs into your daily routine from Day 1. These herbs are key to supporting your liver, kidneys, and digestive system as they start processing and eliminating toxins. Herbal teas and tinctures will help ease digestion, reduce inflammation, and provide gentle detoxification without overwhelming the system (we'll dive into specific herbal rituals below).

4. Eat Light, Easy-to-Digest Meals

In the first five days, focus on consuming lighter, easy-to-digest meals that won't overload your system. Soups, smoothies, and salads made with whole, nutrient-dense ingredients will support your body as it adjusts to the cleanse. Avoid heavy, fried, or overly rich foods that could strain your digestive system during this early phase.

- Opt for steamed vegetables, nourishing broths, and simple grains like quinoa or brown rice paired with plenty of fresh, leafy greens.

By easing into the cleanse, you'll help your body transition more smoothly, allowing it to gradually adapt to the detox process without overwhelming your system or triggering intense detox symptoms.

Daily Herbal Detox Rituals: Teas, Tinctures, and Smoothies That Cleanse and Nourish
Establishing daily herbal detox rituals is an essential part of resetting your digestive system. The herbs you use in these first five days will gently support your liver, kidneys, and digestive tract, promoting detoxification while also nourishing your body. These daily rituals help set the tone for the rest of the cleanse, grounding your body in healing routines that will continue throughout the 15 days.

Here are some **key herbal detox rituals** to incorporate during Days 1-5:

1. Morning Detox Tea

Start each morning with a detox tea to stimulate digestion and support liver detoxification. **Dandelion root** and **milk thistle** are excellent choices for morning detox teas as they help the liver process and eliminate toxins. You can also add lemon, ginger, or turmeric for additional anti-inflammatory benefits.

- **Recipe:** Combine 1 tsp of dandelion root, 1 tsp of milk thistle seeds, and a slice of fresh ginger in hot water. Let it steep for 5-10 minutes and sip slowly to start your day.

2. Mid-Morning Herbal Tinctures

Incorporating herbal tinctures in the middle of the day is a quick and effective way to deliver concentrated doses of detox-supporting herbs to your system. **Burdock root, licorice root,** and **turmeric tinctures** can help with inflammation, digestion, and toxin removal.

- Add 20-30 drops of herbal tincture to a glass of water or tea and consume mid-morning for additional digestive support.

3. Afternoon Smoothies

Smoothies are a great way to pack in essential nutrients, fiber, and detoxifying herbs. For an afternoon boost, create smoothies using fiber-rich fruits, vegetables, and detox herbs like **spirulina, chlorella,** or **turmeric.** These superfoods support detox while giving your body the energy it needs to keep going throughout the day.

- **Recipe:** Blend 1 cup of spinach, 1 banana, 1 tbsp of flaxseeds, ½ cup of frozen berries, 1 tsp of spirulina, and 1 cup of water or almond milk.

4. Evening Herbal Tea

At the end of the day, unwind with a soothing tea that supports digestion and prepares your body for a restful night's sleep. **Peppermint, chamomile,** and **slippery elm** are excellent choices for evening teas that help calm the digestive system and reduce any discomfort from the detox process.

- **Recipe:** Combine 1 tsp of peppermint leaves with 1 tsp of slippery elm bark in hot water. Steep for 5-10 minutes and enjoy before bed.

By establishing these daily herbal rituals, you'll support your body's detox processes while also nourishing it with the vitamins, minerals, and antioxidants it needs to function optimally.

Dealing with Detox Symptoms: What's Normal, What's Not, and How to Stay on Track
As your body begins to detox, it's normal to experience some mild detox symptoms in the first few days. These are often referred to as healing crises, and while they can be uncomfortable, they are a sign that your body is eliminating toxins. However, it's important to know what symptoms are normal and how to manage them so you can stay on track.

Normal Detox Symptoms

These symptoms typically arise due to the release of stored toxins into the bloodstream, where they are processed for elimination. Common symptoms include:

- **Headaches:** As your body reduces its reliance on caffeine, sugar, and processed foods, it's normal to experience mild headaches. Drinking plenty of water and herbal teas can help flush out toxins and reduce discomfort.
- **Fatigue:** Your body is working hard to eliminate toxins, and this can sometimes lead to feelings of tiredness or low energy. Ensure you're getting enough rest and eating nutrient-dense foods to support your energy levels.

- **Digestive Upset:** Bloating, gas, or changes in bowel movements (such as increased frequency) are common as your body adjusts to the increased fiber and detox herbs. These symptoms usually resolve by the end of the first week.

Managing Detox Symptoms

- **Stay Hydrated:** Drink plenty of water, herbal teas, and coconut water to flush out toxins and stay hydrated.
- **Rest:** Listen to your body and get plenty of sleep. Rest allows your body to focus its energy on detoxification and healing.
- **Gentle Movement:** Light exercise, such as walking or yoga, can help stimulate digestion and circulation, which aids in toxin elimination.

What's Not Normal

While mild detox symptoms are common, it's important to pay attention to your body and recognize when something may be off. If you experience severe symptoms such as extreme dizziness, nausea, vomiting, or severe fatigue that persists, it's essential to slow down and possibly consult a healthcare professional. Detoxing should not cause extreme discomfort or disrupt your daily life.

Fiber and Fermentation: The Foods That Help Reset Your Gut Flora

Resetting your gut flora is one of the most important goals of the first phase of the cleanse. Incorporating **fiber** and **fermented foods** during these early days will help promote the growth of beneficial bacteria in your gut and support healthy digestion. Fiber helps sweep out waste and toxins, while fermented foods introduce probiotics that restore balance to your gut microbiome.

Fiber-Rich Foods

Fiber is essential for supporting digestion and promoting regular bowel movements. As you increase your fiber intake, you'll help clear out toxins and improve gut motility, which is crucial during detox.

- **Leafy Greens:** Spinach, kale, and Swiss chard are excellent sources of fiber and chlorophyll, which helps detoxify the liver.
- **Cruciferous Vegetables:** Broccoli, Brussels sprouts, and cauliflower are rich in fiber and sulfur-containing compounds that support liver detoxification.
- **Whole Grains and Seeds:** Quinoa, flaxseeds, and chia seeds provide fiber and essential fatty acids that help regulate digestion and reduce inflammation.

Fermented Foods

Fermented foods are rich in probiotics, which help restore balance to the gut microbiome by promoting the growth of beneficial bacteria. This is particularly important after the gut has been exposed to toxins, processed foods, or antibiotics.

- **Sauerkraut:** Rich in probiotics and fiber, sauerkraut supports gut health and aids digestion.
- **Kimchi:** A spicy fermented vegetable dish that promotes healthy digestion and delivers a variety of beneficial bacteria to the gut.
- **Kefir:** A fermented dairy product (or non-dairy alternative) that is packed with probiotics to support a healthy microbiome.

Incorporating these fiber-rich and fermented foods into your meals during the first five days will help reset your gut flora, promoting better digestion and long-term gut health.

The first five days of the **15-Day Herbal Gut Reset** are all about laying a strong foundation for the cleanse by gently easing your body into the process. By incorporating daily herbal detox rituals, managing detox symptoms effectively, and focusing on fiber and fermented foods, you'll help reset your digestive system and prepare your gut for the deeper detoxification and healing that will follow in the next phases of the cleanse. With the right mindset and preparation, these initial days will set the tone for a successful and transformative detox journey.

Chapter 7:
Days 6-10: Deep Cleansing and Rebuilding

As you move into **Days 6-10** of the **15-Day Herbal Gut Reset,** your body is now entering the deeper stages of detoxification and healing. The initial adjustments from the first five days—such as reduced bloating, increased bowel movements, and a gradual improvement in energy—have prepared your system for the more intensive work that lies ahead. During this phase, the focus shifts to reducing inflammation, rebuilding the gut lining, restoring balance to the microbiome, and maintaining proper hydration to support the body's detox processes.

This chapter covers how to target inflammation using anti-inflammatory herbs, the importance of probiotic-packed meals, the role of hydration in enhancing detoxification, and how to track your progress in digestion, energy, and overall health.

Targeting Inflammation: Using Anti-Inflammatory Herbs to Heal the Gut Lining

By the time you reach Days 6-10, your body has begun the process of flushing out toxins, but now it's time to address inflammation, particularly in the gut. Chronic inflammation is often at the root of many digestive issues and can lead to conditions like **leaky gut syndrome,** where the integrity of the gut lining is compromised. The toxins, processed foods, and stress that your body has been exposed to over time can weaken the gut lining, allowing harmful substances to pass through into the bloodstream, triggering immune responses and systemic inflammation.

In this phase of the cleanse, **anti-inflammatory herbs** play a crucial role in healing the gut lining and reducing overall inflammation in the body. These herbs not only soothe irritated tissues but also promote regeneration of the gut lining, restoring its barrier function and protecting against further damage.

Here are some of the key **anti-inflammatory herbs** you'll use during Days 6-10:

1. Turmeric

Turmeric is one of the most potent anti-inflammatory herbs available. Its active compound, **curcumin,** has been extensively studied for its ability to reduce inflammation in the gut and other areas of the body. Curcumin works by inhibiting pro-inflammatory molecules like **cytokines** and **COX-2,** which contribute to inflammation and pain.

- **How to Use:** Incorporate turmeric into your daily meals by adding it to soups, stews, or smoothies. You can also take turmeric supplements, but make sure they include **black pepper extract,** as this enhances curcumin absorption.

2. Ginger

Ginger is another powerful anti-inflammatory herb that supports digestion and helps reduce bloating, gas, and nausea. Ginger contains compounds called **gingerols** that have been shown to lower inflammation and support the healing of the gut lining.

- **How to Use:** Drink ginger tea daily or add fresh ginger to your meals, smoothies, or juices to promote healing and soothe the digestive tract.

3. Licorice Root

Licorice root is particularly effective in healing the gut lining because it stimulates the production of mucus, which protects the digestive tract from further irritation. It also has anti-inflammatory properties that reduce swelling and discomfort in the gut.

- **How to Use:** Licorice root can be taken in tea or tincture form. Look for **deglycyrrhizinated licorice (DGL),** which is a safer form for long-term use, as it reduces the risk of raising blood pressure.

4. Aloe Vera

Aloe vera has soothing and healing properties that make it ideal for calming inflammation in the digestive tract. It can reduce irritation in the gut lining, promote healing, and support detoxification.

- **How to Use:** Aloe vera juice is an excellent way to incorporate this herb into your detox. Drink a small amount (about 1/4 cup) of aloe vera juice before meals to support gut healing.

By incorporating these herbs into your daily routine during Days 6-10, you'll actively target inflammation, heal the gut lining, and create an environment where your digestive system can function optimally.

Probiotic-Packed Meals: How to Incorporate Fermented Foods for Maximum Benefit
As your body detoxifies and begins to heal the gut, it's critical to restore balance to the microbiome—the community of bacteria that lives in your digestive tract. A healthy gut microbiome is essential for proper digestion, nutrient absorption, and immune function. One of the best ways to restore balance to your gut flora during this phase of the cleanse is by incorporating probiotic-packed meals.

Probiotics are beneficial bacteria that help repopulate your gut with healthy microbes, displacing harmful bacteria and promoting overall gut health. These bacteria play a crucial role in breaking down food, producing vitamins, and regulating the immune system.

Here's how to incorporate **fermented foods** into your cleanse for maximum probiotic benefit:

1. Sauerkraut

Sauerkraut, made from fermented cabbage, is rich in probiotics that help replenish your gut flora. It's also high in fiber, which supports digestion and helps regulate bowel movements.

- **How to Use:** Add a small serving (about 2 tablespoons) of sauerkraut to your meals daily. It pairs well with salads, grains, or roasted vegetables. Be sure to choose raw, unpasteurized sauerkraut to ensure it contains live probiotics.

2. Kimchi

Kimchi is a spicy fermented vegetable dish, usually made with cabbage and radishes. Like sauerkraut, kimchi is packed with probiotics and beneficial enzymes that support digestion.

- **How to Use:** Enjoy a small portion of kimchi as a side dish with your main meals. Its spicy flavor can enhance stir-fries, grain bowls, or even simple salads.

3. Kefir

Kefir is a fermented dairy product that contains a broad range of probiotic strains. It has a tangy flavor and can be consumed as a drink or used as a base for smoothies. Kefir is also available in non-dairy varieties, such as coconut or almond kefir.

- **How to Use:** Drink a small glass (about 1/2 cup) of kefir each day to boost your probiotic intake. You can also blend it into smoothies for added nutrients and probiotics.

4. Miso

Miso is a fermented soybean paste that is rich in probiotics, enzymes, and nutrients. It has been used for centuries in Asian cuisine to promote gut health and digestion.

- **How to Use:** Incorporate miso into soups, salad dressings, or sauces. Miso soup is an easy and delicious way to add probiotics to your diet.

By adding these fermented foods to your meals, you'll enhance the diversity and strength of your gut microbiome, supporting digestion and boosting your immune system during the cleanse.

Supporting Detox with Hydration: How Proper Hydration Enhances Cleansing
Hydration is one of the most important yet often overlooked aspects of a successful detox. During Days 6-10, as your body works harder to eliminate toxins and heal the gut, staying hydrated will be critical to ensuring smooth digestion, efficient toxin removal, and overall well-being.

Here's how **hydration enhances detoxification:**

1. Flushing Out Toxins

As your liver, kidneys, and digestive system work to eliminate toxins, water acts as a medium that helps transport waste products out of the body. Without adequate hydration, toxins can accumulate, leading to fatigue, headaches, and sluggish digestion.

- **Tip:** Aim for at least 8-10 glasses of water per day, and increase this amount if you're physically active or sweating. Herbal teas and broths can also contribute to your daily fluid intake.

2. Supporting Kidney Function

The kidneys play a crucial role in filtering waste and toxins from the blood. Proper hydration ensures that the kidneys function efficiently and helps prevent the buildup of harmful substances. Staying hydrated also reduces the risk of developing kidney stones, which can occur if toxins are concentrated in the urine.

- **Tip:** Drink water infused with **lemon, cucumber,** or **mint** to support kidney function and add a refreshing flavor to your hydration routine.

3. Maintaining Electrolyte Balance

During detoxification, especially when incorporating herbal diuretics like **dandelion root** or **parsley,** your body may lose electrolytes such as sodium, potassium, and magnesium. These minerals are essential for maintaining fluid balance, nerve function, and muscle contractions.

- **Tip:** Replenish electrolytes by drinking coconut water or adding a pinch of **Himalayan salt** to your water. You can also include mineral-rich foods like leafy greens, bananas, and avocados to maintain electrolyte balance.

4. Preventing Constipation

Adequate water intake helps soften stool and promotes regular bowel movements, which are essential for flushing out toxins during a cleanse. Dehydration can lead to constipation, making it harder for your body to eliminate waste effectively.

- **Tip:** Combine hydration with fiber-rich foods like chia seeds, flaxseeds, and leafy greens to promote smooth digestion and prevent constipation.

Staying properly hydrated during Days 6-10 will enhance the detoxification process and support your overall health as your body works to remove toxins and rebuild the gut.

Tracking Progress: Monitoring Changes in Digestion, Energy, and Immune Health
As you reach the midpoint of the cleanse, it's important to take stock of the changes happening in your body. While everyone's detox journey is different, monitoring your progress can help you stay motivated and ensure that the cleanse is working effectively.

Here's what to look for as you **track your progress** in digestion, energy, and immune health:

1. Digestive Health

By this stage, you should notice improvements in digestion, including:

- **Reduced Bloating:** As your gut heals and the microbiome begins to rebalance, you should experience less bloating and gas.
- **Regular Bowel Movements:** Your fiber intake and hydration should promote more regular and complete bowel movements, which are key to toxin elimination.
- **Less Digestive Discomfort:** Any symptoms of indigestion, heartburn, or cramping should start to diminish as your digestive system heals.

2. Energy Levels

As toxins are flushed from your system and your gut starts absorbing nutrients more efficiently, your energy levels should begin to rise. Look for signs of increased vitality, such as:

- **Sustained Energy Throughout the Day:** You may find that you no longer experience mid-afternoon slumps or energy crashes.
- **Mental Clarity:** Improved digestion often leads to clearer thinking and better focus, as your brain benefits from a healthier gut-brain connection.

3. Immune Health

The gut plays a critical role in immune function, and as it heals, you should notice improvements in your immune health:

- **Fewer Illnesses:** If you're someone who frequently gets colds or infections, you may notice a reduction in these symptoms as your immune system strengthens.
- **Reduced Inflammation:** Inflammation-related issues like joint pain, skin flare-ups, or allergies may start to subside as your body's inflammatory response is calmed.

4. Emotional and Mental Well-Being

A healthy gut is closely linked to emotional health, and by now, you may notice improvements in your mood and mental state. Feelings of anxiety, irritability, or brain fog may start to lift as your body becomes less burdened by toxins and inflammation.

During **Days 6-10,** you are moving beyond the initial reset and into the deeper stages of detoxification and rebuilding. By targeting inflammation with powerful herbs, incorporating probiotic-rich meals, staying hydrated, and tracking your progress, you are actively supporting your body's ability to cleanse and heal. This phase is crucial for restoring gut health, strengthening the immune system, and enhancing your overall well-being. Stay committed, as the benefits of your cleanse will continue to unfold in the final days of this journey.

Chapter 8:
Days 11-15: Revitalizing and Strengthening Your Gut

As you enter the final phase of the **15-Day Herbal Gut Reset,** your body has already undergone significant detoxification and healing. By now, you should be feeling lighter, more energized, and experiencing better digestion. However, the final five days of the cleanse are critical for consolidating those gains and setting the foundation for long-term gut health and overall well-being.

In this phase, the focus shifts to **revitalizing and strengthening** your gut, with an emphasis on balancing your microbiome, introducing prebiotic-rich foods, and reinforcing immune function. Additionally, staying motivated and developing post-cleanse strategies are crucial to maintaining the progress you've made. Let's dive into how to ensure a smooth transition and lasting benefits as you complete the cleanse.

Flora Balance: How to Maintain a Healthy Microbiome Post-Cleanse

The health of your **gut microbiome**—the community of trillions of bacteria, viruses, fungi, and other microorganisms living in your digestive tract—plays a critical role in your overall well-being. During the cleanse, you've been actively working to detoxify your system, reduce inflammation, and rebuild your gut lining. But to sustain these benefits post-cleanse, it's important to maintain a balanced microbiome.

Here's how you can continue to support a healthy **flora balance** after the cleanse:

1. Continue Incorporating Probiotics

Probiotics are the beneficial bacteria that help restore balance to the gut microbiome. While you've already included fermented foods like sauerkraut, kimchi, and kefir during the cleanse, it's important to continue consuming these probiotic-rich foods even after the cleanse is over. These foods help maintain a thriving population of good bacteria in your gut, which supports digestion, enhances nutrient absorption, and boosts your immune system.

- **Key Probiotic Foods to Include:** Fermented vegetables (sauerkraut, kimchi), fermented dairy (yogurt, kefir), miso, tempeh, and probiotic supplements if needed.

2. Avoid Processed Foods and Sugar

Processed foods, refined sugars, and artificial additives are some of the biggest culprits when it comes to disrupting gut flora. Harmful bacteria and yeast strains like **Candida** thrive on sugar and processed foods, leading to dysbiosis, an imbalance in the microbiome. To maintain the healthy balance you've cultivated during the cleanse, it's crucial to continue avoiding these inflammatory foods as much as possible.

- **Focus on Whole Foods:** Continue eating a diet rich in fruits, vegetables, whole grains, lean proteins, and healthy fats to nourish your microbiome and keep harmful bacteria in check.

3. Eat a Diverse Diet

One of the most effective ways to maintain a healthy microbiome is to eat a **diverse diet** that provides a wide range of nutrients. Different strains of beneficial bacteria thrive on different types of fibers and plant compounds, so the more varied your diet, the more diverse and robust your gut flora will be. Aim to eat a variety of fruits, vegetables, grains, legumes, and herbs each week.

- **Variety is Key:** Rotate your sources of plant-based foods, such as different types of leafy greens, root vegetables, berries, nuts, seeds, and legumes.

Maintaining a balanced microbiome post-cleanse is essential for long-term gut health. A healthy microbiome not only supports digestion but also plays a crucial role in regulating the immune system, mental health, and overall vitality.

Introducing Prebiotic Foods: Nourishing Your Gut Bacteria for Long-Term Health

While probiotics introduce beneficial bacteria into your gut, **prebiotics** are the fibers and compounds that feed these good bacteria, helping them grow and thrive. Including prebiotic foods in your diet post-cleanse is essential for maintaining the balance of your gut flora and ensuring that the good bacteria can flourish.

Here are some key **prebiotic foods** to incorporate for long-term gut health:

1. Chicory Root

Chicory root is one of the richest sources of **inulin,** a type of prebiotic fiber that supports the growth of beneficial bacteria, particularly **Bifidobacteria.** Inulin helps improve digestion, regulate bowel movements, and enhance nutrient absorption.

- **How to Use:** Chicory root can be brewed as a tea or coffee substitute. You can also find chicory root extract or inulin powder, which can be added to smoothies, baked goods, or oatmeal.

2. Garlic and Onions

Garlic and onions contain **fructooligosaccharides (FOS),** a type of prebiotic fiber that promotes the growth of healthy bacteria in the gut. These foods also have antimicrobial properties that help keep harmful bacteria in check, while nourishing the beneficial strains.

- **How to Use:** Incorporate raw or lightly cooked garlic and onions into your meals, such as salads, stir-fries, or roasted vegetables.

3. Asparagus

Asparagus is a great source of **prebiotic fiber** and helps support digestion by feeding the good bacteria in your gut. It's also rich in antioxidants, which help reduce inflammation and support overall gut health.

- **How to Use:** Steam or roast asparagus and add it to salads, grain bowls, or as a side dish with meals.

4. Bananas

Bananas, particularly when slightly green, contain **resistant starch,** a type of prebiotic that feeds beneficial bacteria in the gut. Resistant starch passes through the small intestine undigested and ferments in the colon, where it promotes the growth of healthy bacteria.

- **How to Use:** Enjoy bananas on their own, in smoothies, or sliced over oatmeal or yogurt. Opt for slightly underripe bananas for the most prebiotic benefit.

5. Flaxseeds

Flaxseeds are a rich source of **fiber** and **lignans,** both of which support the growth of healthy gut bacteria. Flaxseeds also provide omega-3 fatty acids, which have anti-inflammatory properties that support gut health.

- **How to Use:** Add ground flaxseeds to smoothies, oatmeal, or salads for an easy boost of fiber and prebiotics.

By including these prebiotic-rich foods in your post-cleanse diet, you'll ensure that the beneficial bacteria in your gut are well-nourished and able to thrive, supporting long-term digestive health and resilience.

Rebuilding Immune Function: How Detoxing Strengthens Immunity Over Time
A healthy gut is the foundation of a strong immune system, and by detoxifying your body and restoring balance to your gut microbiome, you've already taken significant steps toward strengthening your immune function. During Days 11-15, as your body continues to heal and rebuild, your immune system will also experience long-term benefits from the detox.

Here's how detoxing helps **rebuild and strengthen immunity** over time:

1. Reducing Chronic Inflammation

Chronic inflammation, often caused by poor diet, toxins, and gut dysbiosis, weakens the immune system and makes the body more susceptible to illness and infection. By detoxifying the body and removing inflammatory triggers, you've helped reduce the overall inflammatory load on your immune system. This allows your immune cells to function more efficiently, improving your body's ability to fight off infections and diseases.

- **Long-Term Benefits:** Reduced risk of autoimmune conditions, fewer colds or infections, and improved recovery times from illness.

2. Restoring Gut Integrity

A compromised gut lining can allow harmful substances to leak into the bloodstream, triggering immune responses and leading to chronic immune activation. The healing process you've undergone during the cleanse has helped restore the integrity of your gut lining, reducing the likelihood of **leaky gut syndrome** and preventing unnecessary immune system activation.

- **Long-Term Benefits:** Less immune system overactivity, reduced allergies or sensitivities, and overall stronger immune defense.

3. Balancing Gut Flora

As we've discussed, your gut microbiome plays a critical role in regulating your immune system. By rebalancing your gut flora during the cleanse, you've supported the development of a diverse and healthy microbial population. Beneficial bacteria in the gut help train the immune system to distinguish between harmful invaders and harmless substances, improving immune tolerance and reducing the risk of autoimmune diseases.

- **Long-Term Benefits:** Improved immune regulation, reduced risk of autoimmune disorders, and enhanced ability to ward off infections.

4. Supporting Detoxification Pathways

Your body's detoxification systems—primarily the liver, kidneys, and lymphatic system—play a vital role in maintaining a healthy immune response. By supporting these pathways during the cleanse, you've helped your body more efficiently process and eliminate toxins, reducing the burden on your immune system and improving its overall function.

- **Long-Term Benefits:** A more efficient detox system means your immune system won't be overburdened by toxin exposure, allowing it to focus on protecting your body from pathogens.

As you continue to nourish your gut and support detoxification, your immune system will become stronger and more resilient, providing long-lasting protection against illness and disease.

Staying Motivated: Encouragement for the Final Stretch and Post-Cleanse Strategies
As you approach the end of your cleanse, it's important to stay motivated and focused on your long-term health goals. The last few days of the cleanse are an opportunity to solidify the progress you've made and set yourself up for lasting success. Here's how to stay motivated during the final stretch and beyond:

1. Reflect on Your Progress

Take some time to reflect on how far you've come during the cleanse. Whether it's improved digestion, clearer skin, more energy, or a stronger sense of well-being, acknowledge the positive changes you've experienced. Writing down your progress in a journal can help reinforce your motivation and keep you focused on maintaining these benefits.

- **Tip:** Make a list of the improvements you've noticed in your body, mind, and overall health. Use this as a reminder of the powerful effects of the cleanse.

2. Set New Health Goals

As you prepare to transition out of the cleanse, think about your long-term health goals. Whether it's continuing to focus on gut health, improving your fitness routine, or adopting healthier eating habits, setting new goals will help you stay on track and maintain your momentum.

- **Tip:** Break your goals down into actionable steps, such as continuing to eat more whole foods, incorporating a daily herbal tea ritual, or committing to regular exercise.

3. Create a Post-Cleanse Plan

Once the cleanse is complete, it's important to have a post-cleanse plan in place. This will help you transition back to a more flexible diet without losing the progress you've made. A gradual transition is key—don't rush back to processed foods, sugar, or other inflammatory triggers.

- **Tip:** Continue eating whole, nutrient-dense foods, incorporate probiotics and prebiotics, and maintain hydration. If you reintroduce any foods that were eliminated during the cleanse, do so slowly to monitor how your body responds.

4. Celebrate Your Success

Completing a cleanse is a major accomplishment, and it's important to celebrate your success. Reward yourself for the hard work and dedication you've put into improving your health—whether it's through a relaxing self-care ritual, treating yourself to a favorite healthy meal, or simply taking time to reflect on your journey.

- **Tip:** Plan a fun, health-focused activity to celebrate, such as a cooking class, yoga session, or a nature hike that allows you to enjoy your revitalized energy and well-being.

As you finish Days 11-15, you are entering the most rewarding phase of the **15-Day Herbal Gut Reset.** The hard work of detoxifying, healing, and rebuilding your gut is paying off, and you've laid a strong foundation for lasting health and vitality. By focusing on maintaining flora balance, incorporating prebiotic foods, supporting your immune system, and staying motivated, you'll ensure that the benefits of this cleanse extend well beyond these 15 days.

The journey doesn't end here—this is just the beginning of a healthier, more balanced life. Stay committed to your well-being, continue nourishing your gut, and embrace the positive changes you've achieved.

Part 4: Life After the Cleanse: Maintaining Gut and Immune Health

Chapter 9:
Post-Cleanse: Transitioning Back to Normal Life

Completing the **15-Day Herbal Gut Reset** is a major accomplishment, and by now, your body has gone through significant detoxification, healing, and restoration. However, the work doesn't stop here. The post-cleanse phase is just as important as the cleanse itself because this is where you transition back into your regular lifestyle. How you reintroduce foods, maintain the progress you've made, and continue supporting your body will determine whether the benefits of the cleanse last long-term.

In this chapter, we'll explore how to gradually reintroduce foods, apply the **80/20 rule** for maintaining a healthy gut without being too restrictive, and identify which herbs to continue using for ongoing support. These strategies will help you avoid digestive shock, sustain your gut health, and ensure that your post-cleanse life is balanced and fulfilling.

Reintroducing Foods Gradually: How to Avoid Digestive Shock Post-Cleanse

After spending 15 days on a highly focused cleanse, where you've eliminated certain foods and introduced a variety of gut-supporting herbs and nutrient-dense meals, it can be tempting to jump right back into your previous eating habits. However, doing so too quickly can lead to **digestive shock,** undoing some of the progress you've made during the cleanse. The key is to reintroduce foods gradually, paying close attention to how your body responds.

Why Gradual Reintroduction Matters

During the cleanse, your digestive system has had time to heal, inflammation has been reduced, and your gut microbiome has become more balanced. Reintroducing foods too quickly—especially those that may be inflammatory or difficult to digest—can overwhelm your gut, causing bloating, gas, indigestion, or even flare-ups of previous symptoms.

By gradually reintroducing foods, you give your digestive system time to adjust and can identify any potential food sensitivities or intolerances that may have been masked before the cleanse. This mindful approach helps you maintain the benefits of the cleanse and avoid digestive discomfort.

Steps for Gradually Reintroducing Foods

Here's a step-by-step guide to help you reintroduce foods gradually while monitoring your body's responses:

1. Reintroduce One Food Group at a Time

Rather than bringing back multiple food groups at once, start by reintroducing one food group at a time over the course of 3-4 days. This will allow you to observe how your body reacts to each group and identify any foods that cause discomfort.

- **Start with Whole Grains:** If you eliminated grains during the cleanse, start by reintroducing whole grains like quinoa, brown rice, or oats. These grains are generally easier to digest and are rich in fiber, which supports gut health.
- **Next, Introduce Dairy:** If you tolerate dairy, begin with fermented dairy products like yogurt or kefir, as they contain probiotics that support the gut microbiome. Monitor for any signs of bloating, gas, or discomfort.
- **Then, Introduce Animal Proteins:** If you eliminated animal proteins during the cleanse, reintroduce lean sources like chicken, turkey, or fish. Start with small portions and avoid processed meats, which can be inflammatory.

2. Monitor Your Body's Responses

After reintroducing a food group, pay close attention to how your body responds over the next few days. Keep a food journal where you can track any symptoms like bloating, gas, digestive discomfort, or changes in energy levels. If a certain food group causes negative symptoms, consider eliminating it again for a longer period to allow your gut more time to heal.

3. Avoid Reintroducing Processed Foods and Sugars

While it's important to transition back to a balanced diet, continue to avoid processed foods, refined sugars, and artificial additives as much as possible. These foods can quickly undo the progress you've made during the cleanse by disrupting your gut microbiome and triggering inflammation.

By taking a gradual, mindful approach to reintroducing foods, you'll protect your gut health and avoid overwhelming your digestive system, ensuring that the benefits of the cleanse remain intact.

The 80/20 Rule for Gut Health: Maintaining a Healthy Gut Without Being Restrictive

One of the most common concerns after completing a cleanse is how to maintain the results without becoming overly restrictive or feeling deprived. The 80/20 rule for gut health offers a balanced approach that allows you to enjoy your favorite foods while still prioritizing gut health and maintaining the progress you've made during the cleanse.

What Is the 80/20 Rule?

The 80/20 rule is a simple and flexible guideline for maintaining a healthy lifestyle without being overly rigid. It suggests that **80% of your diet** should consist of nutrient-dense, gut-supporting whole foods, while **20%** of your diet can include more indulgent or less "clean" foods. This balance ensures that you're consistently nourishing your gut with the foods it needs to stay healthy, while also allowing room for occasional treats or meals that may not be as health-focused.

How to Apply the 80/20 Rule to Gut Health

By following the 80/20 rule, you can maintain a healthy gut without feeling restricted or falling into the all-or-nothing mindset that often leads to burnout. Here's how to make the 80/20 rule work for you:

1. Focus on Whole, Gut-Friendly Foods 80% of the Time

Incorporate gut-friendly foods into the majority of your meals. These include:

- **Probiotic-Rich Foods:** Fermented foods like sauerkraut, kimchi, yogurt, kefir, and miso.
- **Prebiotic Foods:** Fiber-rich foods that feed your gut bacteria, such as garlic, onions, leeks, asparagus, and bananas.
- **Anti-Inflammatory Foods:** Leafy greens, berries, fatty fish (rich in omega-3s), and nuts.
- **Whole Grains:** Quinoa, brown rice, oats, and other unprocessed grains that support digestion.
- **Lean Proteins:** Chicken, turkey, fish, legumes, and plant-based proteins.

2. Allow Flexibility 20% of the Time

The remaining 20% of your diet allows for more flexibility. This could include your favorite comfort foods, meals out with friends, or indulging in treats that may not be part of your regular gut health plan. The key is to enjoy these foods mindfully and in moderation, knowing that they won't derail your progress if they're consumed occasionally.

- **Examples of the 20%:** A slice of pizza, a dessert, or a glass of wine on a special occasion.

3. Avoid a Restrictive Mindset

The 80/20 rule is designed to help you maintain a healthy lifestyle without feeling restricted. By allowing room for indulgences, you'll reduce the likelihood of feeling deprived or falling into cycles of bingeing and dieting. This balanced approach promotes long-term sustainability and makes it easier to stick to your gut health goals over time.

By applying the 80/20 rule, you'll maintain a diet that supports your gut health while still allowing for flexibility, making it easier to enjoy your favorite foods without guilt.

Herbal Support After the Cleanse: Which Herbs to Continue for Ongoing Benefits
While the cleanse itself may be complete, continuing to use certain **herbs** can provide ongoing support for your gut, liver, and overall health. Many of the herbs you've incorporated during the **15-Day Herbal Gut Reset** are powerful tools for maintaining long-term health, and continuing to include them in your routine will help protect your body from future toxin buildup and inflammation.

Here are the **key herbs** to continue using post-cleanse for ongoing benefits:

1. Milk Thistle

Milk thistle is a powerful liver-supporting herb that helps detoxify and protect liver cells. As the liver is the body's primary detox organ, supporting its function post-cleanse is essential for maintaining overall health.

- **How to Use:** Take milk thistle in supplement form or drink it as a tea. Consuming milk thistle regularly will help your liver continue processing and eliminating toxins.

2. Turmeric

Turmeric's anti-inflammatory properties make it a valuable herb to continue using after the cleanse. It helps reduce systemic inflammation, supports digestive health, and promotes a healthy immune response.

- **How to Use:** Add turmeric to your meals or take it as a supplement. For better absorption, pair it with black pepper or healthy fats like coconut oil.

3. Ginger

Ginger supports digestion and reduces bloating, making it a great herb to include in your post-cleanse routine. It also has anti-inflammatory properties and can help soothe the digestive tract.

- **How to Use:** Drink ginger tea regularly or add fresh ginger to your meals, smoothies, or juices.

4. Dandelion Root

Dandelion root supports both liver and digestive health. It acts as a mild diuretic, helping the kidneys eliminate waste, and also stimulates bile production, which aids in fat digestion.

- **How to Use:** Continue drinking dandelion root tea or take it in supplement form. It's especially helpful if you plan to indulge in heavier meals or foods that are harder to digest.

5. Slippery Elm

Slippery elm is an excellent herb for soothing the digestive tract and supporting gut healing. It forms a protective coating in the digestive tract, reducing inflammation and promoting healing of the gut lining.

- **How to Use:** Take slippery elm in tea or supplement form if you experience any digestive discomfort or symptoms of indigestion.

By continuing to use these herbs in your daily routine, you'll maintain the progress you've made during the cleanse and provide ongoing support for your digestive system and overall health.

Transitioning back to normal life after the **15-Day Herbal Gut Reset** requires a mindful approach to reintroducing foods, maintaining balance, and continuing to support your body with the tools you've learned during the cleanse. By gradually reintroducing foods, applying the 80/20 rule for long-term gut health, and incorporating key herbs into your daily routine, you'll protect the progress you've made and set yourself up for continued vitality and well-being.

Remember, the post-cleanse phase is not about perfection—it's about balance and sustainability. By embracing these strategies, you'll be able to enjoy the benefits of the cleanse for months and years to come, creating a lifestyle that promotes lasting gut health and overall wellness.

Chapter 10:
Long-Term Gut Health Strategies

Congratulations! By completing the **15-Day Herbal Gut Reset,** you've taken an important step toward revitalizing your gut and laying a foundation for better overall health. However, maintaining the progress you've made and ensuring long-term gut health requires ongoing effort. In this chapter, we'll explore key strategies to integrate into your daily life that will help you maintain a healthy gut for the long haul. By focusing on fiber-rich foods, fermented products, intermittent fasting, probiotics and prebiotics, and an anti-inflammatory diet, you can sustain the benefits of the cleanse and enjoy better digestion, immunity, and well-being.

Fiber, Ferments, and Fasting: Integrating These into Your Everyday Life
Fiber, fermented foods, and **intermittent fasting** are three powerful tools for maintaining gut health and supporting long-term wellness. Each plays a unique role in promoting a healthy digestive system, balancing gut bacteria, and reducing inflammation. Let's take a closer look at how to incorporate these into your everyday life.

1. Fiber: The Foundation of Gut Health

Fiber is essential for healthy digestion and maintaining regular bowel movements. It acts as a "sweeper" in the digestive tract, moving food along and helping eliminate waste. Additionally, fiber feeds the beneficial bacteria in your gut, promoting a healthy microbiome. There are two types of fiber—**soluble** and **insoluble**—both of which are important for overall gut health.

- **Soluble Fiber:** This type of fiber dissolves in water to form a gel-like substance, which slows digestion and helps stabilize blood sugar levels. It also supports gut bacteria by fermenting in the colon, providing food for beneficial microbes. Sources of soluble fiber include oats, apples, carrots, and legumes.
- **Insoluble Fiber:** This fiber adds bulk to the stool and helps prevent constipation by promoting regular bowel movements. Insoluble fiber is found in foods like whole grains, nuts, seeds, and the skins of fruits and vegetables.

How to Integrate More Fiber into Your Diet:

- Start your day with a fiber-rich breakfast, such as oatmeal topped with berries, flaxseeds, and a sprinkle of chia seeds.
- Incorporate more **whole grains** into your meals, such as quinoa, brown rice, barley, or whole-wheat bread.
- Snack on fiber-dense foods like raw vegetables, fruits, and nuts.
- Add legumes (lentils, beans, chickpeas) to salads, soups, and stews.

Aim to consume at least **25-35 grams of fiber** per day to support healthy digestion and nourish your gut microbiome.

2. Ferments: Replenishing Beneficial Bacteria

Fermented foods are rich in probiotics—live bacteria that support gut health by replenishing your microbiome and improving digestion. During the fermentation process, beneficial bacteria break down sugars and starches in the food, producing acids that preserve the food and create a healthy environment for good bacteria to thrive.

Key Fermented Foods to Include in Your Diet:

- **Sauerkraut:** Fermented cabbage rich in probiotics that improve gut health and digestion.
- **Kimchi:** A spicy fermented vegetable dish that supports digestive health and boosts immune function.
- **Kefir:** A fermented milk product (also available in non-dairy varieties) loaded with probiotics and beneficial enzymes.
- **Miso:** A fermented soybean paste used in soups and sauces that enhances digestion.
- **Yogurt:** Opt for plain, unsweetened yogurt with live active cultures for a healthy probiotic boost.

How to Integrate Fermented Foods into Your Daily Life:

- Add a spoonful of **sauerkraut** or **kimchi** to your meals, whether it's as a side dish, in sandwiches, or atop grain bowls.
- Start your day with a small glass of **kefir** or add it to your smoothies for a probiotic boost.
- Enjoy a bowl of **miso soup** as a nourishing snack or side dish.
- Incorporate a serving of plain **Greek yogurt** with fruit and seeds as a snack or breakfast option.

Regularly consuming fermented foods ensures that your gut stays populated with beneficial bacteria, which aids in digestion, reduces bloating, and supports immune function.

3. Fasting: Giving Your Gut a Rest

Intermittent fasting, or the practice of cycling between periods of eating and fasting, is another effective strategy for promoting gut health. When you fast, your digestive system gets a break, allowing your gut lining to heal and giving your microbiome time to rebalance. Fasting can also improve gut motility (the movement of food through the digestive tract) and reduce inflammation.

There are various methods of intermittent fasting, but the most common approach is the **16/8 method,** where you fast for 16 hours and eat all your meals within an 8-hour window. Another method is **5:2 fasting,** where you eat normally for five days of the week and significantly reduce your calorie intake for two days.

How to Incorporate Fasting into Your Routine:

Try the **16/8 method,** where you finish your last meal by 7 or 8 PM and then break your fast around 11 AM the next day. This allows for a 16-hour fasting window while still eating a full day's worth of nutritious meals.

On fasting days, focus on staying hydrated by drinking water, herbal teas, and broth.

Avoid over-eating when you break your fast; instead, focus on balanced meals with protein, healthy fats, and fiber.

Fasting gives your digestive system time to rest and reset, improving overall gut health and supporting longevity.

The Power of Probiotics and Prebiotics: Maintaining Flora Balance for the Long Haul
Maintaining a balanced gut microbiome is essential for long-term health. To keep your microbiome thriving, you need both **probiotics** (beneficial bacteria) and **prebiotics** (the food that feeds them). When combined, these form a **synbiotic relationship,** ensuring that your gut flora remains diverse and healthy.

1. Probiotics: The Beneficial Bacteria

Probiotics are live bacteria that can be consumed through fermented foods or supplements. These beneficial microbes help maintain the balance of good and bad bacteria in the gut, preventing dysbiosis (an imbalance in gut bacteria) that can lead to digestive problems, inflammation, and immune dysfunction.

Benefits of Probiotics:

- Enhance digestion and nutrient absorption.
- Reduce bloating and gas.
- Support the immune system by promoting a balanced inflammatory response.
- Help prevent and treat conditions like irritable bowel syndrome (IBS) and diarrhea.

Probiotic-Rich Foods to Include:

- **Sauerkraut, kimchi, kefir, yogurt, miso,** and other fermented foods (as discussed earlier).
- Consider a high-quality **probiotic supplement** if you have difficulty getting enough probiotics through food alone.

2. Prebiotics: The Food for Beneficial Bacteria

Prebiotics are non-digestible fibers that feed the good bacteria in your gut, promoting their growth and activity. They act as fertilizer for your microbiome, helping maintain a balanced population of beneficial microbes.

Common Prebiotic-Rich Foods:

- **Garlic** and **onions:** Rich in **fructooligosaccharides** (FOS), which feed good bacteria.
- **Bananas** (especially green or slightly underripe bananas): **Contain resistant** starch, which ferments in the colon and feeds beneficial bacteria.
- **Asparagus, artichokes,** and **leeks:** High in **inulin,** a powerful prebiotic fiber.
- **Chicory root:** A potent source of inulin that supports gut health and digestion.

How to Maintain Flora Balance with Probiotics and Prebiotics:

- Include a mix of probiotic and prebiotic-rich foods in your daily diet. For example, enjoy a bowl of yogurt (probiotic) with a topping of sliced bananas and flaxseeds (prebiotic).
- Pair fermented foods like **sauerkraut** or **kimchi** with meals containing prebiotic fibers like garlic, onions, or leeks to create a symbiotic effect.

By regularly consuming both probiotics and prebiotics, you can keep your gut microbiome healthy, balanced, and diverse, promoting better digestion, immune function, and overall well-being.

Anti-Inflammatory Eating: How to Keep Inflammation Low Through Your Diet
Chronic inflammation is a major contributor to digestive issues, autoimmune diseases, and other health problems. Fortunately, many of the foods you eat can either increase or reduce inflammation in your body. Adopting an **anti-inflammatory diet** is one of the best ways to protect your gut and maintain long-term health.

The Impact of Inflammation on Gut Health

When your body is in a state of chronic inflammation, the lining of your gut can become damaged, leading to conditions like **leaky gut syndrome.** This can allow toxins and undigested food particles to pass into the bloodstream, triggering an immune response and worsening inflammation. By reducing inflammation through your diet, you can protect the integrity of your gut lining and reduce your risk of chronic health issues.

Foods to Include in an Anti-Inflammatory Diet:

1. Leafy Greens and Colorful Vegetables

Leafy greens (spinach, kale, collard greens) and colorful vegetables (bell peppers, carrots, sweet potatoes) are rich in **antioxidants** and **phytonutrients** that help fight inflammation and support gut health.

- **Tip:** Incorporate a variety of leafy greens and colorful vegetables into your meals each day, aiming for at least 5-7 servings of vegetables per day.

2. Omega-3 Fatty Acids

Omega-3 fatty acids, found in fatty fish like salmon, sardines, and mackerel, as well as in walnuts and flaxseeds, are potent anti-inflammatories. They help reduce inflammation throughout the body, including in the gut, and support heart and brain health.

- **Tip:** Eat fatty fish at least twice a week, or take a high-quality fish oil supplement to ensure adequate omega-3 intake.

3. Berries and Fruits

Berries, especially blueberries, strawberries, and blackberries, are packed with **antioxidants** called **polyphenols**, which have been shown to reduce inflammation and support gut health. Other fruits like oranges, apples, and pears are also beneficial for their fiber content and anti-inflammatory properties.

- **Tip:** Enjoy a handful of berries as a snack, add them to your smoothies, or toss them on top of oatmeal or yogurt.

4. Nuts and Seeds

Nuts (almonds, walnuts) and seeds (flaxseeds, chia seeds) provide healthy fats, fiber, and antioxidants that help reduce inflammation and promote healthy digestion.

- **Tip:** Add a sprinkle of seeds to your salads, yogurt, or smoothies, or enjoy a handful of nuts as a snack.

5. Herbs and Spices

Certain herbs and spices, like **turmeric, ginger,** and **garlic,** are particularly effective at reducing inflammation. Turmeric contains **curcumin,** a powerful anti-inflammatory compound, while ginger has natural compounds that help lower inflammation and support digestion.

- **Tip:** Use turmeric and ginger in your cooking, teas, or smoothies to boost your anti-inflammatory intake.

Foods to Avoid in an Anti-Inflammatory Diet:

1. Refined Carbohydrates and Sugars

Refined carbs (white bread, pastries, processed snacks) and added sugars promote inflammation and feed harmful bacteria in the gut, leading to imbalances in the microbiome.

- **Tip:** Avoid foods with added sugars, and opt for whole grains over refined carbohydrates.

2. Processed Foods and Trans Fats

Highly processed foods, fried foods, and those containing trans fats can increase inflammation and contribute to poor gut health.

- **Tip:** Focus on whole, unprocessed foods, and cook with healthy fats like olive oil and avocado oil.

By adopting an anti-inflammatory diet, you can keep inflammation in check, protect your gut, and reduce your risk of chronic disease, all while supporting long-term gut health.

The strategies outlined in this chapter—focusing on fiber, fermented foods, intermittent fasting, probiotics, prebiotics, and anti-inflammatory eating—are powerful tools for maintaining long-term gut health. These habits, when integrated into your daily routine, will help ensure that the benefits of the **15-Day Herbal Gut Reset** extend well beyond the initial detox. By making these practices a regular part of your life, you can enjoy sustained digestive health, better immunity, reduced inflammation, and an overall sense of well-being for years to come.

Part 5: Herbal Remedies and Recipes for Digestive Health

Chapter 11:
Herbal Spotlight: Key Ingredients for Gut Cleansing

Herbs have been used for centuries to support digestion and detoxification, and they play a central role in promoting gut health. Throughout the **15-Day Herbal Gut Reset,** you've incorporated several key herbs to aid in the cleansing process, reduce inflammation, and support the overall function of your digestive system. These natural remedies are powerful tools for maintaining long-term gut health.

In this chapter, we'll shine a spotlight on the most effective **digestive herbs,** show you how to create your own **probiotic-rich fermented foods,** and provide easy and delicious **prebiotic-packed recipes** that will continue to nourish your gut flora. By using these herbs and ingredients, you can maintain a healthy gut, improve digestion, and support your overall well-being.

Digestive Herbs: What They Are and How They Work

Digestive herbs are natural remedies that help promote healthy digestion, reduce bloating, soothe inflammation, and assist in the detoxification process. These herbs work in a variety of ways: some stimulate bile production, which aids in the digestion of fats; others help relieve gas and bloating by relaxing the muscles of the digestive tract. Many digestive herbs also have anti-inflammatory properties, making them especially useful in healing the gut lining and supporting long-term gut health.

Here are some of the most effective **digestive herbs** you've encountered during the cleanse, and how they work to support your gut:

1. Ginger: The Warming Digestive Aid

Ginger has been used for thousands of years in traditional medicine to aid digestion, soothe nausea, and reduce inflammation. Ginger contains active compounds called **gingerols** and **shogaols,** which stimulate digestion, reduce gas, and relieve bloating. It also helps to speed up the emptying of the stomach, making it useful for those who suffer from indigestion or discomfort after eating.

- **How It Works:** Ginger improves gastric motility, meaning it helps food move more efficiently through the digestive system. It also has antispasmodic properties that relax the muscles in the intestines, reducing cramping and bloating.
- **How to Use:** Drink ginger tea before or after meals, add freshly grated ginger to smoothies and soups, or take ginger supplements if you experience frequent digestive discomfort.

2. Dandelion: The Liver Supporter

Dandelion root is a powerful herb for liver and digestive health. It stimulates the production of bile, which helps the body break down fats and absorb fat-soluble vitamins. Dandelion also acts as a gentle diuretic, supporting the kidneys in the removal of waste and excess water. It's particularly useful in detoxification programs, as it promotes liver health and enhances digestion.

- **How It Works:** Dandelion root supports liver function by increasing bile production, which aids in fat digestion. It also helps cleanse the liver of toxins and supports healthy elimination through the kidneys.
- **How to Use:** Drink dandelion root tea daily or incorporate dandelion root tincture into your herbal routine. You can also use fresh dandelion greens in salads for an extra nutrient boost.

3. Fennel: The Bloat Buster

Fennel is an excellent herb for reducing gas, bloating, and indigestion. It contains compounds that relax the muscles in the digestive tract, allowing trapped gas to pass more easily. Fennel is also mildly anti-inflammatory and helps stimulate the production of digestive enzymes, which improves the breakdown and absorption of nutrients.

- **How It Works:** Fennel seeds contain **anethole**, a compound that reduces inflammation in the digestive tract and eases bloating. It also has carminative properties, meaning it helps prevent the formation of gas in the digestive system.
- **How to Use:** Chew fennel seeds after meals to reduce bloating, or brew fennel tea for digestive support. You can also add fresh fennel to salads or roasted vegetable dishes for a sweet, licorice-like flavor.

4. Peppermint: The Soothing Antispasmodic

Peppermint is another classic herb for soothing digestive discomfort. It has antispasmodic properties, meaning it helps relax the muscles in the digestive tract and reduces cramping and bloating. Peppermint also stimulates bile flow, aiding in the digestion of fats. It's commonly used to treat symptoms of irritable bowel syndrome (IBS), indigestion, and gas.

- **How It Works:** Peppermint oil contains **menthol,** which has a relaxing effect on the smooth muscles of the intestines, helping to relieve bloating, gas, and abdominal discomfort.
- **How to Use:** Drink peppermint tea after meals or use peppermint oil capsules if you suffer from chronic digestive discomfort. Peppermint leaves can also be added to salads or smoothies for a refreshing flavor.

5. Licorice Root: The Gut Healer

Licorice root is known for its soothing and anti-inflammatory properties. It is particularly beneficial for healing the gut lining and reducing inflammation in the digestive tract. Licorice root stimulates the production of mucus, which protects the stomach and intestines from irritation. It is often used to treat conditions like leaky gut syndrome, acid reflux, and ulcers.

- **How It Works:** Licorice root contains **glycyrrhizin,** which helps reduce inflammation and stimulates the production of protective mucus in the gut. This makes it an effective herb for soothing and healing the digestive lining.

- **How to Use:** Drink licorice root tea, or take deglycyrrhizinated licorice (DGL) supplements to soothe inflammation and support gut healing.

Probiotic-Rich Foods: How to Create Your Own Fermented Foods

Fermented foods are packed with probiotics—beneficial bacteria that help restore balance to the gut microbiome and improve digestion. While store-bought fermented foods are a convenient option, making your own fermented foods at home is simple, cost-effective, and allows you to control the quality and ingredients. Creating your own probiotic-rich foods can become a regular part of your long-term gut health strategy.

Here are some popular **fermented foods** you can make at home:

1. Sauerkraut: A Classic Fermented Cabbage

Sauerkraut is one of the easiest fermented foods to make at home. All you need is cabbage, salt, and time. The fermentation process creates an environment where beneficial bacteria thrive, transforming the cabbage into a gut-friendly food rich in probiotics.

Ingredients:

- 1 medium cabbage (green or red)
- 1 tablespoon sea salt
- Optional: Carrots, garlic, or spices for flavor

Instructions:

- Remove the outer leaves of the cabbage, then thinly slice the remaining cabbage.
- Place the sliced cabbage in a large bowl and sprinkle with salt. Massage the cabbage with your hands for about 10 minutes, until it begins to release water.
- Pack the cabbage tightly into a glass jar, pressing down to submerge it in its own liquid. Make sure the cabbage is fully covered by the liquid to prevent mold from forming.
- Cover the jar with a lid or cloth and let it ferment at room temperature for 1-4 weeks, depending on how tangy you like it. Check it regularly and press the cabbage down if needed to keep it submerged.
- Once it reaches your desired level of fermentation, store the sauerkraut in the refrigerator.

2. Kimchi: A Spicy Fermented Vegetable Dish

Kimchi is a traditional Korean dish made from fermented cabbage and other vegetables, flavored with garlic, ginger, chili peppers, and fish sauce. It's rich in probiotics and adds a flavorful kick to your meals.

Ingredients:

- 1 medium napa cabbage
- 2 tablespoons sea salt

- 4 garlic cloves, minced
- 1 tablespoon ginger, minced
- 2 tablespoons chili flakes (adjust for spice level)
- 2 tablespoons fish sauce (optional)
- 1 carrot, julienned

Instructions:

- Cut the cabbage into quarters and soak in salted water for about 2 hours. Rinse and drain well.
- In a separate bowl, mix the garlic, ginger, chili flakes, and fish sauce.
- Toss the cabbage and carrots with the spice mixture, making sure the vegetables are evenly coated.
- Pack the mixture into a glass jar, pressing down to remove any air pockets. Ensure the vegetables are submerged in their own juices.
- Cover and let ferment at room temperature for 3-7 days. Once it reaches your preferred flavor, store in the refrigerator.

3. Kefir: A Probiotic-Rich Fermented Milk Drink

Kefir is a fermented milk product similar to yogurt but with a thinner consistency and a wider range of beneficial bacteria. You can make kefir at home using **kefir grains** (available online or at health food stores) and any type of milk, including non-dairy options like coconut or almond milk.

Ingredients:

- 1 tablespoon kefir grains
- 2 cups milk (dairy or non-dairy)

Instructions:

- Place the kefir grains in a clean glass jar and pour the milk over them.
- Cover the jar loosely with a lid or cloth and let it sit at room temperature for 24-48 hours, depending on the desired thickness and tanginess.
- Strain the kefir to remove the grains (which can be reused for the next batch) and store the kefir in the refrigerator.

These homemade fermented foods are packed with probiotics that help maintain a balanced gut microbiome, improve digestion, and support long-term gut health.

Prebiotic-Packed Recipes: Easy, Delicious Meals to Feed Your Gut Flora

In addition to probiotics, **prebiotics** are essential for feeding your gut flora and promoting the growth of beneficial bacteria. Prebiotics are found in fibrous foods like garlic, onions, leeks, asparagus, bananas, and whole grains. Incorporating prebiotic-rich foods into your diet is a simple and delicious way to nourish your gut microbiome.

Here are a few **prebiotic-packed recipes** to keep your gut flora healthy and thriving:

1. Garlic and Leek Soup

This hearty soup is loaded with prebiotics from garlic, onions, and leeks, making it a perfect meal for supporting your gut health.

Ingredients:

- 4 garlic cloves, minced
- 2 leeks, chopped
- 1 onion, chopped
- 4 cups vegetable broth
- 2 carrots, diced
- 1 tablespoon olive oil
- 1 teaspoon thyme
- Salt and pepper to taste

Instructions:

- In a large pot, heat the olive oil and sauté the garlic, leeks, and onion until softened.
- Add the carrots, thyme, and broth, and bring to a boil.
- Reduce heat and simmer for 20 minutes, until the vegetables are tender.
- Season with salt and pepper, then serve.

2. Banana and Chia Seed Pudding

This simple chia seed pudding is rich in prebiotics from bananas and chia seeds. It makes for a delicious, fiber-packed breakfast or snack.

Ingredients:

- 1 ripe banana
- 3 tablespoons chia seeds
- 1 cup almond milk (or any milk of choice)
- 1 teaspoon vanilla extract
- A pinch of cinnamon

Instructions:

- Mash the banana in a bowl, then stir in the chia seeds, almond milk, vanilla, and cinnamon.
- Let the mixture sit for at least 2 hours (or overnight) in the refrigerator until it thickens.
- Serve chilled, topped with additional banana slices or berries.

3. Roasted Asparagus with Garlic and Lemon

Asparagus is a powerhouse of prebiotics, and this roasted dish is a delicious way to enjoy it.

Ingredients:

- 1 bunch asparagus, trimmed
- 2 garlic cloves, minced
- 1 tablespoon olive oil
- 1 tablespoon lemon juice
- Salt and pepper to taste

Instructions:

- Preheat your oven to 400°F (200°C).
- Toss the asparagus with olive oil, garlic, and lemon juice, then spread it on a baking sheet.
- Roast for 15-20 minutes, until tender and slightly crispy.
- Season with salt and pepper and serve.

You've learned about the power of **digestive herbs,** the benefits of creating your own **fermented foods,** and how to prepare **prebiotic-packed recipes** to feed your gut flora. These tools are essential for maintaining a healthy gut long after the cleanse is over. By continuing to integrate these herbs, probiotics, and prebiotics into your daily life, you'll ensure that your digestive system remains balanced, your microbiome stays healthy, and your overall well-being flourishes. The journey to long-term gut health is ongoing, but with these strategies, you're well-equipped to sustain and even improve the progress you've made.

Chapter 12:
Recipes for Gut Health

Maintaining a healthy gut requires a balanced approach, one that integrates herbal remedies, fermented foods, prebiotic-rich meals, and anti-inflammatory ingredients. With these tools, you can actively support your digestive health while enjoying delicious and nourishing meals. This chapter provides a collection of recipes tailored to promote gut health, featuring soothing **herbal detox teas,** simple **fermented foods,** quick and nutrient-dense **prebiotic smoothies,** and **anti-inflammatory meals** that help heal and soothe the digestive system.

Herbal Detox Teas: Soothing Blends for Daily Use

Herbal detox teas are a gentle and effective way to support digestion, reduce bloating, and detoxify the body. The herbs in these blends work together to soothe the digestive system, stimulate detoxification, and promote the elimination of waste. These teas are easy to prepare and can be enjoyed daily for ongoing gut support.

1. Ginger and Turmeric Detox Tea

This warming tea is a powerful anti-inflammatory blend that soothes the digestive tract and promotes detoxification. **Ginger** stimulates digestion, while **turmeric** provides potent anti-inflammatory benefits, making this tea perfect for daily gut health.

Ingredients:

- 1-inch piece fresh ginger, sliced
- 1 teaspoon turmeric powder (or a 1-inch piece of fresh turmeric, sliced)
- Juice of 1 lemon
- 1 teaspoon honey (optional)
- 2 cups water

Instructions:

- In a small pot, bring the water, ginger, and turmeric to a boil.
- Reduce the heat and simmer for 10 minutes.
- Strain the tea into a mug and stir in the lemon juice and honey (if using).
- Drink warm to soothe digestion and support detoxification.

2. Peppermint and Fennel Tea

This refreshing tea is excellent for reducing bloating and gas. **Peppermint** has antispasmodic properties that help relax the muscles of the digestive tract, while **fennel** aids digestion and reduces bloating by relieving gas.

Ingredients:

- 1 teaspoon dried peppermint leaves (or 1 peppermint tea bag)

- 1 teaspoon fennel seeds
- 2 cups boiling water

Instructions:

- Place the peppermint leaves and fennel seeds in a teapot or mug.
- Pour the boiling water over the herbs and let steep for 5-10 minutes.
- Strain the tea and enjoy it after meals to aid digestion and relieve bloating.

3. Dandelion and Licorice Root Tea

This tea supports liver detoxification and gut healing. **Dandelion root** stimulates bile production, aiding fat digestion, while **licorice root** helps soothe and repair the digestive lining.

Ingredients:

- 1 tablespoon dried dandelion root
- 1 teaspoon licorice root (deglycyrrhizinated, or DGL)
- 2 cups water

Instructions:

- Bring the water to a boil and add the dandelion root and licorice root.
- Reduce heat and simmer for 10 minutes.
- Strain the tea and enjoy it warm, especially after meals to support digestion.

Fermented Foods: Simple Recipes for Homemade Probiotics
Fermented foods are rich in probiotics, which help restore the balance of beneficial bacteria in the gut and improve digestion. Making your own fermented foods at home is simple, cost-effective, and allows you to enjoy fresh, gut-friendly ingredients. Below are a few easy recipes to get started with homemade fermented foods.

1. Classic Sauerkraut

Sauerkraut is one of the simplest and most beneficial fermented foods you can make at home. This recipe requires only two ingredients—cabbage and salt—and provides your gut with a powerful source of probiotics.

Ingredients:

- 1 medium green or red cabbage, finely shredded
- 1 tablespoon sea salt

Instructions:

- Place the shredded cabbage in a large bowl and sprinkle with salt.
- Massage the cabbage with your hands for about 10 minutes, until it begins to release its liquid.

- Pack the cabbage tightly into a large glass jar, pressing it down so that the liquid covers the cabbage completely.
- Cover the jar with a lid or cloth and let it ferment at room temperature for 1-4 weeks, depending on your taste preference.
- Once fermented, store the sauerkraut in the refrigerator and enjoy as a side dish or topping for meals.

2. Easy Kimchi

Kimchi is a spicy, probiotic-rich Korean dish made from fermented vegetables. This easy recipe combines napa cabbage with garlic, ginger, chili flakes, and fish sauce for a flavorful and gut-friendly dish.

Ingredients:

- 1 medium napa cabbage
- 2 tablespoons sea salt
- 4 garlic cloves, minced
- 1 tablespoon ginger, minced
- 2 tablespoons chili flakes
- 2 tablespoons fish sauce (optional)
- 1 carrot, julienned

Instructions:

- Slice the cabbage into quarters and soak in salted water for 2 hours. Drain and rinse.
- In a large bowl, combine garlic, ginger, chili flakes, fish sauce, and carrots.
- Toss the cabbage with the spice mixture, coating it evenly.
- Pack the mixture tightly into a glass jar, ensuring it is submerged in its own juices.
- Let the kimchi ferment at room temperature for 3-7 days, then refrigerate and enjoy as a side dish or condiment.

3. Kefir

Kefir is a fermented milk drink packed with probiotics. It's easy to make at home and can be enjoyed as a drink or added to smoothies for extra gut health benefits.

Ingredients:

- 1 tablespoon kefir grains
- 2 cups milk (dairy or non-dairy)

Instructions:

- Add the kefir grains to a glass jar and pour in the milk.
- Cover the jar loosely and let it ferment at room temperature for 24-48 hours.
- Strain the kefir to remove the grains and store the kefir in the refrigerator.

- The grains can be reused to make another batch of kefir.

Prebiotic Smoothies: Quick and Easy Drinks to Nourish Your Gut Bacteria
Prebiotics are the fibers that feed beneficial bacteria in the gut, helping them thrive. Prebiotic-rich foods include bananas, garlic, onions, and chicory root, among others. These smoothie recipes are packed with prebiotics and are easy to make, making them a perfect way to start your day or enjoy as a healthy snack.

1. Green Banana Prebiotic Smoothie

Bananas, especially when slightly green, are a rich source of resistant starch, which acts as a prebiotic for gut bacteria. This smoothie combines green bananas with leafy greens and seeds for a fiber-packed, gut-nourishing drink.

Ingredients:

- 1 green banana
- 1 cup spinach or kale
- 1 tablespoon chia seeds
- 1 cup almond milk
- 1 teaspoon honey (optional)

Instructions:

- Combine all ingredients in a blender and blend until smooth.
- Enjoy immediately as a refreshing, prebiotic-rich breakfast or snack.

2. Flax and Berry Prebiotic Smoothie

Flaxseeds are an excellent source of fiber and prebiotics, while berries provide antioxidants that support gut health. This smoothie is delicious, easy to prepare, and great for gut bacteria.

Ingredients:

- 1/2 cup frozen mixed berries (blueberries, raspberries, strawberries)
- 1 tablespoon ground flaxseeds
- 1/2 cup plain yogurt or kefir (optional for probiotics)
- 1 cup almond milk
- 1 teaspoon vanilla extract

Instructions:

- Place all ingredients in a blender and blend until smooth.
- Serve chilled, and enjoy this fiber-packed, gut-nourishing smoothie.

3. Chicory Root Prebiotic Latte

Chicory root is a potent prebiotic that helps feed beneficial gut bacteria. This chicory root latte is a delicious alternative to coffee and supports digestive health.

Ingredients:

- 1 tablespoon chicory root powder
- 1 cup hot water
- 1/2 cup almond milk (or other milk of choice)
- 1 teaspoon honey or maple syrup (optional)

Instructions:

- Brew the chicory root powder in hot water as you would coffee.
- Heat the almond milk and froth if desired.
- Combine the chicory root brew with the almond milk and sweeten with honey or maple syrup.
- Enjoy this warm, prebiotic-rich drink.

Anti-Inflammatory Meals: Recipes to Heal and Soothe the Digestive System
An anti-inflammatory diet is key to promoting gut healing, reducing inflammation, and supporting overall health. These meals are packed with ingredients that soothe the digestive system, reduce inflammation, and provide essential nutrients for gut health.

1. Turmeric Lentil Soup

This nourishing soup combines anti-inflammatory ingredients like turmeric, ginger, and garlic with fiber-rich lentils, making it a perfect meal for healing and supporting digestion.

Ingredients:

- 1 cup red lentils, rinsed
- 1 onion, diced
- 2 garlic cloves, minced
- 1 tablespoon grated ginger
- 1 teaspoon turmeric powder
- 1 teaspoon cumin
- 4 cups vegetable broth
- 1 tablespoon olive oil
- Salt and pepper to taste

Instructions:

- In a large pot, heat the olive oil and sauté the onion, garlic, and ginger until softened.
- Add the turmeric and cumin, stirring for 1 minute.

- Pour in the broth and add the lentils. Bring to a boil, then reduce heat and simmer for 20-25 minutes, until the lentils are tender.
- Season with salt and pepper and serve warm.

2. Wild Salmon with Avocado and Quinoa

This anti-inflammatory meal is rich in omega-3 fatty acids from wild salmon, healthy fats from avocado, and fiber from quinoa. It's a nutrient-dense meal that supports gut health and reduces inflammation.

Ingredients:

- 2 wild-caught salmon fillets
- 1 avocado, sliced
- 1 cup cooked quinoa
- 1 tablespoon olive oil
- Juice of 1 lemon
- Salt and pepper to taste

Instructions:

- Preheat the oven to 400°F (200°C).
- Place the salmon fillets on a baking sheet, drizzle with olive oil, and season with salt, pepper, and lemon juice.
- Bake for 12-15 minutes, until the salmon is cooked through.
- Serve the salmon over a bed of quinoa, topped with avocado slices and a drizzle of extra lemon juice.

3. Roasted Sweet Potatoes with Tahini Dressing

Sweet potatoes are packed with anti-inflammatory compounds and are easy to digest. This simple roasted sweet potato dish is paired with a creamy tahini dressing for a delicious and gut-friendly meal.

Ingredients:

- 2 large sweet potatoes, cubed
- 1 tablespoon olive oil
- 1/4 cup tahini
- Juice of 1 lemon
- 1 garlic clove, minced
- 1 tablespoon maple syrup
- Salt and pepper to taste

Instructions:

- Preheat the oven to 425°F (220°C).

- Toss the sweet potatoes with olive oil, salt, and pepper, and spread on a baking sheet.
- Roast for 25-30 minutes, until tender and slightly caramelized.
- In a small bowl, whisk together tahini, lemon juice, garlic, maple syrup, and a bit of water to thin the dressing.
- Drizzle the tahini dressing over the roasted sweet potatoes and serve.

In this chapter, you've gained a variety of delicious and nutritious recipes that will continue to support your gut health long after the cleanse. By regularly incorporating **herbal detox teas, fermented foods, prebiotic-rich smoothies,** and **anti-inflammatory meals** into your diet, you'll not only maintain the benefits of the **15-Day Herbal Gut Reset** but also promote long-term gut health and overall well-being. These recipes are easy to integrate into daily life and will help you build a lifestyle that prioritizes digestion, inflammation control, and a thriving gut microbiome.

Part 6: Overcoming Detox Skepticism and Sticking to the Plan

Chapter 13:
Handling Detox Doubts

Embarking on a detox journey can be both exciting and daunting. While the benefits of cleansing—improved digestion, increased energy, reduced bloating, and enhanced overall wellness—are widely discussed, detox programs often raise questions and doubts. Whether you're new to detoxing or have tried several methods in the past, it's normal to experience uncertainty. This chapter addresses common concerns and misconceptions about detoxing, highlights real-life success stories from people who have experienced profound benefits from detox programs, and provides guidance on how to measure success beyond the scale.

Common Concerns and Misconceptions: Addressing the Most Frequent Questions About Detoxing

Detox programs often come with a mix of skepticism and curiosity. While some people believe in the transformative power of detoxing, others are hesitant, influenced by various misconceptions. Let's debunk some of the most common concerns and clarify what you can truly expect from a well-structured detox like the **15-Day Herbal Gut Reset.**

1. "Detoxing is Just a Trend—Does My Body Really Need It?"

One of the most prevalent misconceptions is that detoxing is just a fad. The human body is equipped with natural detoxification systems (liver, kidneys, skin, and lymphatic system) that work continuously to remove toxins. So, why would we need an additional detox program?

While it's true that the body can detoxify itself, modern lifestyles can overwhelm these systems. Processed foods, environmental pollutants, chemicals, medications, and stress can all place an excessive burden on your detox organs. Over time, this can lead to toxin buildup, sluggish digestion, and inflammation, making it harder for your body to function optimally.

- **Clarification:** A detox program supports your body's natural detox processes by reducing the intake of toxins and providing nutrient-dense, anti-inflammatory foods and herbs that enhance liver function, support digestion, and promote toxin elimination. Rather than being a trend, detoxing is a way to give your body a "reset" in a world filled with environmental and dietary stressors.

2. "Will I Be Hungry All the Time?"

A common fear about detoxing is that you'll be hungry, deprived, or restricted to an extreme diet of juices or fasting. While some detox programs may involve fasting or juice cleanses, the **15-Day Herbal Gut Reset** focuses on **nourishing** your body with real, whole foods and herbs that promote detoxification while keeping you satisfied.

- **Clarification:** The detox includes fiber-rich vegetables, fruits, legumes, lean proteins, healthy fats, and herbs, ensuring that you receive balanced nutrition without feeling hungry. This isn't about deprivation but about eliminating inflammatory foods and replacing them with nutrient-dense options that support gut health.

3. "Will I Experience Uncomfortable Detox Symptoms?"

Detox symptoms such as headaches, fatigue, irritability, or digestive changes can occur as the body begins to release stored toxins. While some discomfort may be experienced, it is typically mild and temporary, especially with proper hydration and gradual easing into the detox.

- **Clarification:** These symptoms are often referred to as "healing crises," where the body is adjusting to the detox process. Symptoms usually subside after a few days. Drinking plenty of water, herbal teas, and consuming fiber-rich foods can help alleviate these effects. Remember, these symptoms are a sign that your body is actively eliminating toxins, and the benefits will follow soon.

4. "Isn't Detoxing Harmful to My Body?"

Some detox programs, especially extreme juice fasts or highly restrictive diets, can put undue stress on the body, leading to nutrient deficiencies or muscle loss. However, a well-structured detox, like the **15-Day Herbal Gut Reset,** is designed to be safe, sustainable, and nourishing.

- **Clarification:** This detox provides all the essential macronutrients (protein, fats, carbohydrates) and micronutrients (vitamins, minerals) your body needs while removing inflammatory foods and adding detox-supporting herbs. The goal is to support your body, not starve it. If you follow the plan as recommended, detoxing is not harmful but rather restorative.

5. "Will I Lose Weight During the Detox?"

Weight loss is often a side effect of detoxing, but it should not be the primary goal. Detoxing focuses on improving digestion, reducing inflammation, and eliminating toxins, which may naturally lead to weight loss as your body becomes more balanced.

- **Clarification:** If weight loss does occur, it's typically due to reduced bloating, improved digestion, and the elimination of processed foods and sugars. However, the more significant outcomes are increased energy, clearer skin, better digestion, and overall improved health.

Real Results, Real People: Case Studies and Testimonials from Previous Users

The best way to overcome doubts about detoxing is by hearing from real people who have experienced the transformative benefits firsthand. The following case studies and testimonials illustrate the power of the **15-Day Herbal Gut Reset** in improving gut health, boosting energy, and enhancing overall wellness.

Case Study 1: Sarah's Journey from Bloating to Balance

Sarah, a 35-year-old marketing professional, had struggled with chronic bloating, fatigue, and digestive discomfort for years. After trying various diets and supplements with little success, she decided to give the **15-Day Herbal Gut Reset** a try.

- **Initial Concerns:** Sarah was skeptical about detoxing, fearing she'd feel hungry or restricted. However, after reading about the focus on whole foods and herbs, she decided to move forward.
- **Detox Experience:** During the first few days, Sarah experienced mild headaches and fatigue, but by Day 5, she noticed a significant reduction in bloating and an increase in energy. By Day 10, her digestion had improved, and she no longer felt sluggish after meals.
- **Results:** By the end of the detox, Sarah had lost 5 pounds of water weight, but more importantly, she felt more balanced, energetic, and free of the bloating that had plagued her for years. Her skin also cleared up, and she continued many of the dietary habits she learned during the detox.

Testimonial: "I can't believe how much better I feel after just 15 days! I no longer experience the bloating that used to make me uncomfortable every day, and I have so much more energy. This detox has changed the way I think about food, and I'm excited to continue these habits in my daily life."

Case Study 2: Jason's Quest for Energy and Mental Clarity

Jason, a 42-year-old entrepreneur, was struggling with brain fog, low energy, and occasional digestive issues. As someone who led a busy lifestyle, he often relied on processed foods and caffeine to get through the day but found himself feeling drained and unfocused.

- **Initial Concerns:** Jason was unsure whether a detox would provide real benefits, as he had never done one before. He was also concerned about finding the time to prepare detox-friendly meals.
- **Detox Experience:** Jason noticed improvements by Day 3, with fewer cravings for sugary snacks and more consistent energy throughout the day. By Day 8, his brain fog had lifted, and he felt more focused and productive.
- **Results:** Jason finished the detox feeling energized, clear-headed, and more in control of his diet. He found that meal preparation was easier than he expected, and he planned to continue incorporating detox-friendly meals into his routine.

Testimonial: "This detox was a game-changer for me. I've never felt this clear-headed or energetic in years. The best part is that I didn't feel deprived—I actually enjoyed the meals and discovered new foods that I'll keep eating long after the detox."

Case Study 3: Emily's Battle with Skin Issues

Emily, a 29-year-old teacher, had dealt with hormonal acne and skin inflammation for most of her adult life. She suspected that her skin issues were connected to her diet and digestion but wasn't sure how to address it. She decided to try the **15-Day Herbal Gut Reset** to see if it could help her skin and digestion.

- **Initial Concerns:** Emily was concerned that the detox wouldn't have a noticeable impact on her skin, as she had tried many topical treatments without success.
- **Detox Experience:** In the first week, Emily noticed that her skin was beginning to clear, and her digestion improved. By the end of the detox, her acne had reduced significantly, and her skin looked healthier overall.
- **Results:** The detox helped Emily identify foods that were triggering her skin issues. She learned how her gut health played a key role in her skin, and by continuing the detox principles, she saw long-lasting improvements in both her skin and digestion.

Testimonial: "I never realized how much my gut health was affecting my skin until I did this detox. My acne has cleared up more in two weeks than it did after years of trying different products. I feel like I finally have control over my health and my skin."

How to Measure Success: Using Non-Scale Victories to Gauge Your Progress
While weight loss may be a benefit of detoxing, it's important to look beyond the scale when measuring your success. Detox programs like the **15-Day Herbal Gut Reset** offer numerous health benefits that may not always be reflected by a number on the scale. These are known as **non-scale victories (NSVs),** and they are critical to understanding the true impact of your detox journey.

1. Improved Digestion and Reduced Bloating

One of the most common benefits of detoxing is improved digestion, which often leads to reduced bloating, more regular bowel movements, and less discomfort after meals. Pay attention to how your body feels after eating—are you less bloated or gassy? Are you experiencing smoother digestion? These are important signs that your detox is working.

2. Increased Energy and Mental Clarity

Another key non-scale victory is an increase in energy levels and mental clarity. Many people experience reduced fatigue, fewer energy crashes, and a clearer mind as their body flushes out toxins and inflammation. If you find that you're more productive, energized, or focused, this is a significant indicator of detox success.

3. Clearer Skin and Reduced Inflammation

Detoxing often improves skin health, as your body eliminates toxins that can contribute to acne, inflammation, and dullness. If your skin is clearer, brighter, or less inflamed, it's a positive sign that your detox is having an impact.

4. Improved Sleep

Detoxing can also improve sleep quality by reducing inflammation, balancing blood sugar levels, and promoting relaxation through the elimination of caffeine and sugar. If you're sleeping more soundly or waking up feeling more refreshed, this is another non-scale victory to celebrate.

5. Emotional Well-Being

Your mental and emotional health can also improve as a result of detoxing. Many people report feeling less stressed, more positive, and more in control of their health after completing a detox program. This sense of emotional well-being is a powerful indicator of long-term success.

Handling detox doubts is an important part of any wellness journey. By addressing common concerns, learning from real-life success stories, and focusing on non-scale victories, you can build confidence in the detox process and fully appreciate the benefits it offers. Whether you're improving digestion, increasing energy, or clearing your skin, detoxing is about creating a healthier, more balanced life. As you continue your journey, remember to celebrate all the positive changes—both big and small—that come with detoxing and caring for your body.

Chapter 14:
Staying Motivated Beyond the Cleanse

Completing the **15-Day Herbal Gut Reset** is a significant achievement, but maintaining the progress you've made requires ongoing commitment. Detoxing has likely provided a boost in energy, clearer skin, better digestion, and improved overall well-being. However, keeping the momentum going after the cleanse can be a challenge, especially when life returns to its usual pace. In this chapter, we'll explore how to stay motivated beyond the cleanse by building a routine that supports long-term digestive health, dealing with setbacks in a productive way, and understanding the connection between self-care, mental well-being, and gut health.

Building a Routine: How to Make Digestive Health a Part of Your Lifestyle

The success of your detox hinges on your ability to make the habits you formed during the cleanse part of your everyday life. Building a routine that supports digestive health doesn't have to be complicated, but it does require intentional planning. By incorporating key practices into your daily routine, you'll be able to maintain the benefits of the cleanse, support your gut, and prevent setbacks.

1. Prioritize Whole Foods in Your Diet

One of the biggest changes you likely made during the cleanse was eliminating processed foods, refined sugars, and artificial ingredients. Continuing to focus on a whole foods diet is essential for maintaining gut health. Whole foods—such as fresh vegetables, fruits, whole grains, lean proteins, and healthy fats—are rich in nutrients and fiber that promote digestion, support the gut microbiome, and reduce inflammation.

- **Tip:** Start your day with a fiber-rich breakfast, such as oatmeal topped with chia seeds, berries, and nuts. Plan meals around vegetables, lean proteins, and whole grains, and keep healthy snacks like fruits, nuts, and prebiotic-rich foods (like garlic and onions) readily available.

2. Establish Regular Mealtimes

Regular mealtimes help regulate your digestion and prevent overeating or snacking on unhealthy foods. Your digestive system functions best when meals are spaced out at consistent intervals, allowing your body to digest food thoroughly between meals. This practice also supports gut motility and helps prevent bloating and indigestion.

- **Tip:** Eat three balanced meals each day at regular times, and avoid eating late at night. If you find yourself needing a snack between meals, opt for a gut-friendly choice like a handful of almonds or a slice of avocado toast on whole-grain bread.

3. Stay Hydrated

Proper hydration is critical for maintaining digestive health. Water helps break down food, aids in nutrient absorption, and supports bowel movements by preventing constipation. During the cleanse, you likely focused on drinking more water and herbal teas—this is a habit to continue post-cleanse.

- **Tip:** Drink 8-10 glasses of water per day, and add herbal teas like peppermint, ginger, or dandelion root to support digestion. You can also add lemon or cucumber slices to your water for a refreshing twist.

4. Incorporate Movement into Your Daily Routine

Exercise and physical activity stimulate digestion by promoting healthy gut motility and reducing stress. Movement encourages regular bowel movements, helps reduce bloating, and supports overall digestive health. Even gentle exercises like walking or yoga can make a difference.

- **Tip:** Aim for at least 30 minutes of physical activity each day. This could include a morning walk, an after-dinner yoga session, or strength training at the gym. If you're pressed for time, even 10-15 minutes of movement can help keep your digestion on track.

5. Practice Mindful Eating

During the cleanse, you likely became more mindful of what you were eating and how it made you feel. Continuing to practice mindful eating helps prevent overeating, improves digestion, and allows you to be more in tune with your body's hunger and fullness cues.

- **Tip:** Take the time to sit down and eat without distractions (like your phone or TV). Chew your food thoroughly, savor each bite, and listen to your body's signals to stop eating when you're full. This will improve digestion and help you feel more satisfied after meals.

Dealing with Setbacks: How to Recover if You Slip Up During the Cleanse

Setbacks are a natural part of any health journey, and they're bound to happen at some point. Whether it's indulging in a sugary treat, eating processed foods during a busy week, or skipping a workout, it's important to approach these moments with compassion and resilience. The key to long-term success is knowing how to recover from setbacks without letting them derail your progress entirely.

1. Accept That Setbacks Happen

The first step in dealing with a setback is acknowledging that it's a normal part of the journey. No one eats perfectly all the time, and life's demands can sometimes get in the way of your health goals. The important thing is to avoid guilt or negative self-talk, as these can make you feel discouraged and more likely to give up.

- **Tip:** When you slip up, take a moment to reflect on what led to the setback. Were you stressed, tired, or rushed? By identifying the trigger, you can develop strategies to prevent similar setbacks in the future. Remember that progress isn't linear, and every day is an opportunity to make healthier choices.

2. Get Back on Track with Your Next Meal

One of the most common mistakes people make after a setback is adopting an "all-or-nothing" mentality. For example, indulging in a sugary dessert might lead to thinking, "I've ruined my diet, so I might as well keep eating poorly." Instead of falling into this trap, focus on getting back on track with your next meal.

- **Tip:** If you have a setback, don't wait until tomorrow or next week to start eating healthy again. Plan your next meal around nutrient-dense, gut-friendly foods like a salad with leafy greens, roasted vegetables, and lean protein. This will help you reset and refocus without prolonging the setback.

3. Revisit Your Why

When motivation starts to wane, it's helpful to reconnect with the reasons you embarked on the cleanse in the first place. What were your initial goals? Whether it was to improve your digestion, increase your energy, clear your skin, or reduce inflammation, revisiting your "why" can reignite your motivation and remind you of the benefits you've already experienced.

- **Tip:** Keep a journal of your detox journey, and include both your initial goals and the progress you've made. When setbacks happen, revisit your journal to remind yourself of why you started and how far you've come.

4. Make a Plan for Future Setbacks

Preventing future setbacks requires a plan. Think about what challenges you might face in maintaining your healthy habits and how you can overcome them. Whether it's planning meals ahead of time, preparing snacks for busy days, or finding stress-management techniques, having a strategy in place will help you stay on track.

- **Tip:** Create a list of healthy go-to meals and snacks that are easy to prepare when you're short on time. Keep your kitchen stocked with these items so you always have healthy options available, even during hectic days.

Self-Care and Gut Health: How Mental and Emotional Wellness Influence Digestion

The connection between the mind and the gut is well established. The gut is often referred to as the "second brain" because it has its own nervous system, the **enteric nervous system,** which communicates with the brain and plays a key role in regulating digestion. When you're stressed, anxious, or emotionally drained, your digestive system often bears the brunt, leading to symptoms like bloating, indigestion, or even gut dysbiosis. Therefore, taking care of your mental and emotional well-being is just as important as eating the right foods for your gut.

1. The Gut-Brain Axis: How Stress Affects Digestion

The **gut-brain axis** is the communication network that links your gut and brain. When you experience stress or emotional upset, your brain sends signals to your gut that can disrupt normal digestion. This can lead to a variety of digestive symptoms, including stomach pain, constipation, diarrhea, and bloating. Chronic stress can also contribute to inflammation in the gut and disrupt the balance of your gut microbiome.

- **Tip:** Managing stress is critical for maintaining gut health. Incorporate stress-reduction techniques like deep breathing, meditation, or yoga into your daily routine to support both your mental health and digestion.

2. Prioritize Rest and Sleep

Lack of sleep and overexertion can negatively affect your gut health by increasing stress hormones like cortisol, which contribute to inflammation. Sleep is a restorative time for your body and plays an important role in regulating digestion and gut motility. Poor sleep can also lead to overeating or cravings for unhealthy foods, further disrupting your gut health.

- **Tip:** Aim for 7-9 hours of quality sleep each night. Create a relaxing bedtime routine that includes winding down at least 30 minutes before bed, turning off screens, and engaging in calming activities like reading or stretching. This will improve both your mental well-being and your digestion.

3. Practice Self-Compassion and Mindfulness

Self-compassion is essential for maintaining long-term motivation and overcoming setbacks. When you approach your health journey with kindness and understanding, rather than harsh criticism, you're more likely to stick with your goals and make sustainable changes. Mindfulness practices, such as meditation and mindful eating, can also help you tune into your body's needs, reduce stress, and improve digestion.

- **Tip:** Spend a few minutes each day practicing mindfulness. This could be a short meditation session, deep breathing exercises, or simply taking time to reflect on your progress and what you're grateful for. These practices help you stay grounded, reduce stress, and enhance your overall well-being.

4. Build a Support System

Staying motivated beyond the cleanse is much easier when you have a support system in place. Whether it's friends, family, or a community of like-minded individuals, having people who share your goals and support your journey can make a significant difference. They can provide encouragement during setbacks, celebrate your progress, and help you stay accountable.

- **Tip:** Share your goals with a trusted friend or join a community focused on health and wellness. Regular check-ins, whether in person or online, can help keep you motivated and provide a sense of accountability.

Staying motivated beyond the **15-Day Herbal Gut Reset** requires a combination of planning, self-compassion, and an understanding of the mind-gut connection. By building a routine that supports long-term digestive health, knowing how to handle setbacks without derailing your progress, and prioritizing self-care practices that reduce stress and promote mental well-being, you'll be well-equipped to maintain the benefits of the cleanse. Your health journey doesn't end with the detox—it's an ongoing process of learning, adapting, and nourishing both your body and mind for sustained wellness.

Conclusion:
Your Gut Health Journey Starts Now

As you reach the end of the **15-Day Herbal Gut Reset,** it's important to recognize that this is not the end of your journey—it's just the beginning. You've taken a significant step toward better health by committing to this cleanse, and now it's time to build on the progress you've made. The gut plays a central role in overall health and well-being, and by prioritizing your digestive system, you've unlocked the potential for long-term vitality, resilience, and balance.

In this conclusion, we'll explore why gut health is the cornerstone of wellness, how to maintain the benefits of the cleanse over the long term, and why your path forward should be one of confidence, self-compassion, and continued learning. Your gut health journey truly starts now, and with the right knowledge and mindset, you'll be able to thrive for years to come.

The Power of Gut Health: Why a Healthy Gut Is the Key to Overall Wellness

The gut is often called the "second brain," but its influence extends far beyond digestion. A healthy gut is essential for many aspects of your physical, mental, and emotional well-being. From digestion and nutrient absorption to immune function and even mood regulation, the gut is at the center of it all. Understanding the profound impact that your gut has on your body can motivate you to prioritize its health long after the cleanse is over.

1. Gut Health and Digestion

At its core, the digestive system is responsible for breaking down food, absorbing nutrients, and eliminating waste. When your gut is healthy, these processes work efficiently, ensuring that your body gets the nutrients it needs to function optimally. A balanced gut microbiome helps regulate digestion, reduce bloating, and prevent issues like constipation, diarrhea, or indigestion.

- **Key takeaway:** Maintaining a healthy gut ensures smooth digestion, better nutrient absorption, and fewer digestive disturbances, which in turn supports your energy levels and overall vitality.

2. Gut Health and Immunity

A significant portion of your immune system resides in your gut—up to 70% of your immune cells are located in the gut lining. A healthy, balanced microbiome plays a crucial role in protecting the body from harmful pathogens, regulating inflammation, and training the immune system to distinguish between harmful invaders and harmless substances. When your gut is balanced, your immune system becomes more resilient.

- **Key takeaway:** By supporting your gut health, you strengthen your immune system, helping your body ward off illness, fight infections, and maintain a balanced inflammatory response.

3. Gut Health and Mental Well-Being

The connection between your gut and brain, known as the **gut-brain axis,** underscores how much your digestive health influences your mental well-being. The gut produces neurotransmitters such as **serotonin,** often called the "feel-good" hormone, which regulates mood, sleep, and appetite. When your gut is healthy, you're more likely to experience mental clarity, reduced anxiety, and improved mood. Conversely, an imbalanced gut can contribute to brain fog, stress, and even depression.

- **Key takeaway:** A healthy gut not only supports digestion but also plays a vital role in emotional and mental health. By prioritizing gut health, you can experience greater emotional balance, better sleep, and improved cognitive function.

4. Gut Health and Inflammation

Chronic inflammation is a common issue linked to poor gut health. Processed foods, sugar, environmental toxins, and stress can all contribute to an imbalanced microbiome and inflammation in the gut lining. This can lead to leaky gut syndrome, where harmful substances escape into the bloodstream, triggering an immune response. By reducing inflammation through a gut-healthy diet, you can protect your body from inflammatory diseases, reduce joint pain, improve skin conditions, and support cardiovascular health.

- **Key takeaway:** Gut health is key to reducing systemic inflammation, which is associated with a range of chronic conditions from autoimmune diseases to cardiovascular issues.

Understanding the power of gut health highlights why taking care of your digestive system is the foundation for achieving long-term wellness. By keeping your gut in balance, you're supporting nearly every function in your body, from digestion and immunity to mood and inflammation control.

Staying the Course: How to Maintain the Benefits of Your 15-Day Cleanse Long Term

The **15-Day Herbal Gut Reset** has given you a fresh start, but maintaining these benefits requires ongoing effort and commitment. The good news is that the habits you've formed during the cleanse—such as eating whole, nutrient-dense foods, staying hydrated, and incorporating herbs into your routine—can easily become a part of your everyday life.

1. Continue Eating Whole Foods

One of the biggest takeaways from the cleanse is the importance of a whole foods diet. Processed foods, refined sugars, and artificial additives disrupt your gut microbiome and contribute to inflammation. To maintain the benefits of the cleanse, continue to prioritize vegetables, fruits, whole grains, lean proteins, and healthy fats in your diet. These foods nourish your gut, support digestion, and provide the fiber and nutrients necessary for gut health.

- **Tip:** Make meal planning a weekly habit. Prepare large batches of whole food meals, such as roasted vegetables, quinoa, and lean proteins, so you always have healthy options on hand.

2. Keep Hydrating

Staying hydrated is essential for digestion and detoxification. Water helps move food through your digestive system, supports nutrient absorption, and prevents constipation. Herbal teas can also provide ongoing benefits by soothing digestion and reducing inflammation.

- **Tip:** Aim to drink 8-10 glasses of water each day, and incorporate herbal teas like peppermint, ginger, and chamomile into your routine for added digestive support.

3. Incorporate Probiotic and Prebiotic Foods

Supporting your gut microbiome is crucial for maintaining long-term gut health. Probiotic-rich foods like sauerkraut, kimchi, kefir, and yogurt introduce beneficial bacteria into your gut, while prebiotic foods like garlic, onions, leeks, and bananas feed those bacteria, helping them thrive.

- **Tip:** Include fermented foods in at least one meal a day and add prebiotic-rich vegetables to your salads, soups, and smoothies to keep your gut flora balanced.

4. Manage Stress

As you learned during the cleanse, the gut-brain connection plays a critical role in digestion and overall well-being. Stress can wreak havoc on your gut health by disrupting the balance of bacteria and increasing inflammation. To maintain the benefits of the cleanse, incorporate stress-management practices into your routine.

- **Tip:** Practice daily mindfulness, meditation, or deep breathing exercises to reduce stress. Physical activity, yoga, or even spending time in nature can also help lower stress levels and support gut health.

5. Make Movement a Daily Habit

Regular physical activity supports digestion by stimulating gut motility, reducing bloating, and relieving constipation. Exercise also helps reduce inflammation and supports overall well-being. Whether you prefer walking, swimming, yoga, or strength training, aim to move your body every day.

- **Tip:** Start with 20-30 minutes of exercise each day. This could include a morning walk, yoga, or a strength-training session. Choose activities you enjoy so that exercise becomes a sustainable part of your lifestyle.

6. Use Herbs for Ongoing Support

Herbs such as ginger, turmeric, peppermint, and dandelion are powerful allies for gut health. They support digestion, reduce inflammation, and promote detoxification. Incorporating these herbs into your daily routine will help maintain the progress you made during the cleanse.

- **Tip:** Continue drinking herbal detox teas or add fresh herbs to your meals. You can also use herbal supplements, such as milk thistle for liver support or licorice root for gut healing, to enhance your overall digestive health.

By staying the course and incorporating these habits into your daily routine, you'll be able to maintain the benefits of the cleanse and continue to support your gut health for the long term.

Your Path Forward: Encouraging Readers to Continue Their Wellness Journey with Confidence

Now that you've completed the cleanse and learned how to prioritize gut health, the next step is to move forward with confidence. You've gained the knowledge, tools, and experience necessary to take control of your health and well-being. Your wellness journey doesn't end here—it's a lifelong process of listening to your body, making informed choices, and adapting as you learn more about what works best for you.

1. Trust Your Body's Signals

One of the most valuable lessons from the cleanse is learning how to listen to your body's signals. Whether it's recognizing when you're hungry or full, noticing how certain foods affect your digestion, or paying attention to how stress impacts your gut, tuning in to these signals will help you make better decisions for your health.

- **Encouragement:** Trust your body's wisdom. If certain foods or habits make you feel energized and balanced, continue to incorporate them into your routine. If something doesn't feel right, adjust and experiment with new approaches. Your body will guide you toward the habits that support your long-term well-being.

2. Continue Learning

Health is a journey, not a destination. As you continue along your wellness path, remain open to learning more about your body, gut health, and overall wellness. Whether it's through reading, research, or experimenting with new foods and practices, continuing your education will help you stay informed and empowered.

- **Encouragement:** Stay curious about your health. Read books on nutrition and wellness, attend workshops, and explore new recipes and self-care practices. Knowledge is power, and the more you learn, the more confident you'll feel in making decisions that support your health.

3. Be Kind to Yourself

Self-compassion is essential for staying motivated and making long-term changes. There will be days when you slip up, skip a workout, or indulge in foods that aren't gut-friendly—and that's okay. What matters is how you respond to those moments. By approaching setbacks with kindness and understanding, you'll be more likely to get back on track and continue moving forward.

- **Encouragement:** Practice self-compassion. Your health journey will have ups and downs, but every small step you take toward better health counts. Celebrate your progress, forgive yourself when things don't go as planned, and always focus on what you can do today to support your body.

4. Embrace a Balanced Approach

True health is about balance, not perfection. Your gut health journey should enhance your life, not restrict it. By following the 80/20 rule, you can enjoy your favorite indulgences while still maintaining a healthy diet and lifestyle most of the time. This balance will help you stay consistent and prevent burnout.

- **Encouragement:** Embrace balance. Enjoy the foods you love in moderation, prioritize your mental and emotional well-being, and stay active in a way that feels good to you. Health is about finding what works for you and making it sustainable for the long term.

Your Gut Health Journey Starts Now

You've completed the **15-Day Herbal Gut Reset,** and you've gained valuable insights into how your gut health impacts your entire body. Now, it's time to take this knowledge and apply it to your everyday life. By continuing to nourish your gut, practice self-care, and stay motivated, you'll not only maintain the benefits of the cleanse but also unlock the potential for a healthier, more balanced life.

Your gut health journey starts now, and with the tools, habits, and confidence you've gained, you're well-equipped to continue this journey with success. Remember, the path to health is ongoing—stay curious, stay compassionate, and most importantly, stay committed to your well-being. Your gut—and your body—will thank you for it.

Bonuses

Bonus 1: 7-Day Pre-Cleanse Preparation Guide

7-Day Pre-Cleanse Preparation Guide: Preparing for Success

Before diving into the **15-Day Herbal Gut Reset,** it's important to lay a strong foundation by preparing your body, mind, and kitchen for the detox. The **7-Day Pre-Cleanse Preparation Guide** is designed to help you gradually transition into the cleanse by eliminating common inflammatory foods, establishing healthy habits, and setting realistic expectations for the journey ahead. This pre-cleanse phase will not only make the detox more effective but will also minimize detox symptoms like fatigue, headaches, or cravings.

The focus during this pre-cleanse week is to gently reduce the intake of processed foods, sugars, caffeine, and alcohol while increasing your consumption of whole, nutrient-dense foods and herbal teas. By the time you start the 15-day cleanse, your body will be better equipped to handle the detox process, and you'll feel more prepared mentally and physically.

Why Pre-Cleanse Preparation Is Essential

The pre-cleanse phase allows your body to gradually adjust to the upcoming detox. Jumping straight into a cleanse without preparation can lead to uncomfortable detox symptoms, such as headaches, irritability, fatigue, and digestive upset. By easing into the process, you give your body time to adapt, reduce your toxic load, and stabilize energy levels, making the transition into the detox smoother and more sustainable.

Benefits of a Pre-Cleanse Week:

- **Reduced Detox Symptoms:** A gradual reduction of toxins helps minimize the intensity of detox symptoms.
- **Improved Digestion:** Your digestive system begins to reset before the full detox, allowing for better nutrient absorption and elimination.
- **Increased Energy Levels:** Easing into whole foods and reducing processed foods helps stabilize blood sugar levels and improve energy.
- **Mental Clarity:** By eliminating foods and substances that cause brain fog, such as sugar and caffeine, you'll begin to experience clearer thinking and better focus.
- **Emotional Preparedness:** The pre-cleanse helps set realistic expectations and builds motivation for the full 15-day cleanse.

Pre-Cleanse Week Overview

Over the next seven days, you'll gradually transition away from inflammatory and processed foods and introduce more whole, plant-based meals, herbal teas, and hydration. The pre-cleanse week is broken down into daily goals that help ease you into the full detox.

Day 1-2: Start Cutting Back on Processed Foods and Sugars

Goals for Days 1-2:

- **Eliminate Processed Foods:** Begin reducing your intake of packaged and processed foods, including chips, cookies, frozen meals, and fast food. These foods are often high in artificial ingredients, preservatives, and unhealthy fats that burden your digestive system and contribute to inflammation.
- **Reduce Sugary Beverages and Sweets:** Eliminate sugary drinks like sodas, fruit juices, and sweetened coffees. Gradually reduce your intake of refined sugars found in candies, pastries, and desserts.
- **Hydrate:** Aim for at least 8-10 glasses of water per day. Proper hydration supports digestion, flushes out toxins, and prepares your body for detox.

Sample Meals for Days 1-2:

- **Breakfast:** A bowl of oatmeal topped with fresh berries, chia seeds, and a drizzle of honey or almond butter.
- **Lunch:** A large salad with mixed greens, avocado, cucumbers, tomatoes, and a protein source (chicken, tofu, or beans). Drizzle with olive oil and lemon juice for dressing.
- **Dinner:** Grilled salmon or roasted vegetables (carrots, zucchini, and sweet potatoes) with a side of quinoa or brown rice.
- **Snacks:** Fresh fruits like apples, oranges, or a handful of almonds.

Tip: Pay attention to food labels. Avoid foods with added sugars, artificial sweeteners, and trans fats. Focus on whole, unprocessed ingredients.

Day 3-4: Reduce Caffeine and Alcohol Intake

Goals for Days 3-4:

- **Begin Weaning Off Caffeine:** Start by reducing your daily caffeine intake if you typically consume coffee, energy drinks, or sodas. Try replacing one cup of coffee with an herbal tea (like peppermint or chamomile) or a green tea (which has lower caffeine content) to avoid withdrawal symptoms like headaches and irritability.
- **Eliminate Alcohol:** Alcohol places stress on the liver, which will be a primary detox organ during the cleanse. Eliminate all alcoholic beverages to give your liver a break and prepare for detox.
- **Increase Fiber Intake:** Incorporate more fiber-rich foods, such as vegetables, fruits, legumes, and whole grains, to support digestion and bowel regularity.

Sample Meals for Days 3-4:

- **Breakfast:** A green smoothie made with spinach, banana, chia seeds, almond milk, and a teaspoon of flaxseed oil.

- **Lunch:** A quinoa and black bean salad with cilantro, avocado, cherry tomatoes, and lime dressing.
- **Dinner:** Stir-fried tofu or chicken with broccoli, bell peppers, and brown rice. Season with ginger and garlic.
- **Snacks:** Raw vegetables (carrot sticks, cucumber slices) with hummus or a handful of walnuts.

Tip: If you experience caffeine withdrawal symptoms like headaches, ensure you stay hydrated, and consider taking short breaks to rest as your body adjusts.

Day 5: Increase Plant-Based Meals

Goals for Day 5:

- **Go Plant-Based for the Day:** Shift the focus of your meals to plant-based ingredients for at least one day during the pre-cleanse week. This helps your digestive system reset, providing it with the fiber, vitamins, and minerals it needs to detoxify efficiently.
- **Incorporate Prebiotics and Probiotics:** Add prebiotic-rich foods like garlic, onions, leeks, and asparagus, which feed healthy gut bacteria. Incorporate probiotic foods like yogurt, sauerkraut, and kefir to start balancing your gut microbiome before the full cleanse.
- **Stay Hydrated:** Continue drinking plenty of water, and add detox-supporting herbal teas like dandelion root or ginger to your hydration routine.

Sample Meals for Day 5:

- **Breakfast:** Chia pudding made with almond milk, topped with fresh berries and a sprinkle of cinnamon.
- **Lunch:** Lentil and vegetable soup with kale, carrots, celery, and garlic.
- **Dinner:** Roasted sweet potatoes and brussels sprouts, served with a mixed greens salad and avocado.
- **Snacks:** A bowl of sauerkraut or a serving of plain Greek yogurt with flaxseeds.

Tip: Focus on fiber-rich, anti-inflammatory ingredients to promote digestion and prepare your gut for the cleanse.

Day 6: Prepare Mentally and Organize Your Kitchen

Goals for Day 6:

- **Mindset Preparation:** Take time today to mentally prepare for the detox. Reflect on your goals, and set intentions for the cleanse. Use journaling or meditation to connect with your motivation and visualize the benefits of completing the detox.
- **Stock Your Kitchen:** Clean out your pantry and refrigerator by removing any processed or sugary foods that could tempt you during the cleanse. Stock up on fresh vegetables,

fruits, whole grains, and herbs that you'll need for the upcoming 15 days. Organize your kitchen to make it easier to prepare healthy meals.

- **Meal Prep:** Prepare and pre-cook a few simple meals like roasted vegetables, quinoa, or soups that will save you time during the first few days of the cleanse.

Sample Meals for Day 6:

- **Breakfast:** Overnight oats with chia seeds, almond milk, and fresh fruit.
- **Lunch:** Vegetable stir-fry with tofu or tempeh, served with a side of brown rice.
- **Dinner:** Cauliflower and chickpea curry with turmeric, served over a bed of spinach.
- **Snacks:** Sliced apples with almond butter or raw carrots and cucumber with a tahini dip.

Tip: Create a shopping list for the cleanse. Include detox-friendly foods like leafy greens, lemons, garlic, turmeric, ginger, and herbal teas. Meal planning will help you stay on track during the cleanse.

Day 7: Final Preparations and Setting Realistic Expectations

Goals for Day 7:

- **Visualize Your Success:** Spend time today visualizing yourself completing the 15-day cleanse successfully. Imagine how you'll feel—lighter, more energized, less bloated, and with better digestion. Visualizing positive outcomes helps you stay motivated when challenges arise.
- **Set Realistic Expectations:** Understand that detoxing is a journey. Some days will be easier than others, and you may experience moments of discomfort as your body releases toxins. Remind yourself that these symptoms are temporary and part of the healing process.
- **Herbal Tea Focus:** Begin drinking herbal detox teas that will support you throughout the cleanse. Try a combination of dandelion root (for liver support), ginger (for digestion), and peppermint (to ease bloating).

Sample Meals for Day 7:

- **Breakfast:** A smoothie bowl made with frozen berries, spinach, almond butter, and a sprinkle of hemp seeds.
- **Lunch:** A hearty salad with mixed greens, beets, walnuts, and a lemon-tahini dressing.
- **Dinner:** Roasted butternut squash and sautéed kale, served with lentils.
- **Snacks:** A handful of sunflower seeds or a probiotic-rich kombucha drink.

Tip: Create a space in your home where you can relax, meditate, and practice self-care during the cleanse. This will be a place for mental rejuvenation and reflection.

Entering the Cleanse with Confidence

By following this **7-Day Pre-Cleanse Preparation Guide,** you've set yourself up for a successful detox experience. You've gradually reduced your intake of processed foods, sugars, caffeine, and alcohol, while increasing your consumption of whole, plant-based meals, fiber, and herbal teas. You've taken the time to mentally and physically prepare for the cleanse, organized your kitchen, and stocked up on gut-friendly foods.

Now, you're ready to embark on the **15-Day Herbal Gut Reset** with confidence and enthusiasm, knowing that your body is primed for detoxification and healing. Keep this pre-cleanse preparation guide as a resource to return to whenever you need a reset or want to start another cleanse in the future.

Bonus 2: Post-Cleanse Recipe Book: 30 Gut-Friendly Meals for Long-Term Health

Post-Cleanse Recipe Book: 30 Gut-Friendly Meals for Long-Term Health

Congratulations on completing the **15-Day Herbal Gut Reset!** As you move forward from the cleanse, it's essential to maintain the progress you've made by continuing to nourish your body with wholesome, gut-friendly meals. This **Post-Cleanse Recipe Book** provides 30 delicious, easy-to-prepare meals that support digestion, reduce inflammation, and help maintain a balanced gut microbiome.

These recipes are designed to provide a wide range of essential nutrients, fibers, probiotics, and prebiotics that support long-term gut health. They incorporate anti-inflammatory foods, fiber-rich ingredients, and probiotic-packed fermented foods to keep your digestive system functioning optimally and prevent the recurrence of gut issues.

This guide will offer:

- **Breakfasts** to energize your day and support healthy digestion.
- **Lunches** that are light yet filling, featuring fiber and prebiotic-rich ingredients.
- **Dinners** packed with nutrients and anti-inflammatory ingredients to support gut healing.
- **Snacks** and **Sides** that provide additional nutrition between meals, including probiotic and prebiotic-rich options.
- **Fermented Food Recipes** to help you easily incorporate homemade probiotics into your diet.

Breakfast Recipes

Starting your day with a gut-friendly breakfast helps set the tone for improved digestion and sustained energy throughout the day. These breakfasts are rich in fiber, probiotics, and essential nutrients, promoting a healthy microbiome and balanced energy levels.

1. Chia Seed Pudding with Berries and Almond Butter

Chia seeds are a fantastic source of fiber and omega-3 fatty acids, both of which are essential for gut health. The added almond butter provides healthy fats, while the berries offer antioxidants.

Ingredients:

- 3 tablespoons chia seeds
- 1 cup almond milk (or any plant-based milk)
- 1 teaspoon vanilla extract
- 1 tablespoon almond butter
- 1/2 cup mixed berries
- A drizzle of honey or maple syrup (optional)

Instructions:

- Mix the chia seeds, almond milk, and vanilla extract in a bowl. Let it sit for at least 4 hours or overnight in the fridge.
- Top with almond butter, berries, and a drizzle of honey or maple syrup before serving.

2. Gut-Healing Green Smoothie

This smoothie is packed with gut-friendly ingredients like spinach, avocado, and flaxseeds. Spinach is a great source of prebiotic fiber, while avocado provides healthy fats that soothe inflammation.

Ingredients:

- 1 cup spinach
- 1/2 avocado
- 1 tablespoon flaxseeds
- 1/2 frozen banana
- 1 cup unsweetened almond milk
- 1 teaspoon honey (optional)

Instructions:

- Combine all ingredients in a blender and blend until smooth.
- Serve immediately and enjoy this fiber-packed, anti-inflammatory smoothie.

3. Oatmeal with Flaxseeds, Almonds, and Blueberries

Oatmeal is a prebiotic-rich food that promotes the growth of beneficial gut bacteria. This recipe adds flaxseeds for additional fiber and omega-3s, as well as blueberries for antioxidants.

Ingredients:

- 1/2 cup rolled oats
- 1 tablespoon ground flaxseeds
- 1 tablespoon almond butter
- 1/2 cup blueberries
- 1 cup water or almond milk

Instructions:

- Cook the oats in water or almond milk according to the package instructions.
- Stir in the ground flaxseeds and almond butter.
- Top with blueberries before serving.

Lunch Recipes

Lunches in this recipe book are designed to be light yet filling, helping you maintain energy levels and supporting digestion throughout the day. These meals incorporate fiber-rich vegetables, lean proteins, and healthy fats to keep your gut functioning optimally.

4. Quinoa Salad with Avocado, Spinach, and Sunflower Seeds

Quinoa is a complete protein and a great source of fiber, which supports digestion. This salad is balanced with healthy fats from avocado and seeds, making it a perfect light meal for gut health.

Ingredients:

- 1/2 cup cooked quinoa
- 1 cup spinach
- 1/2 avocado, diced
- 1 tablespoon sunflower seeds
- 1 tablespoon olive oil
- Juice of 1 lemon
- Salt and pepper to taste

Instructions:

- Combine the quinoa, spinach, avocado, and sunflower seeds in a bowl.
- Drizzle with olive oil and lemon juice, then season with salt and pepper.
- Toss well and serve.

5. Lentil and Vegetable Soup

This hearty soup is packed with fiber from lentils and vegetables, making it perfect for promoting gut motility and preventing bloating.

Ingredients:

- 1 cup lentils, rinsed
- 2 carrots, chopped
- 2 celery stalks, chopped
- 1 onion, diced
- 2 garlic cloves, minced
- 4 cups vegetable broth
- 1 teaspoon turmeric
- Salt and pepper to taste

Instructions:

- Sauté the onions, garlic, carrots, and celery in olive oil until softened.
- Add the lentils, vegetable broth, and turmeric.

- Bring to a boil, then reduce heat and simmer for 20-25 minutes until the lentils are tender. Season with salt and pepper before serving.

6. Chickpea and Kale Salad with Lemon-Tahini Dressing

Chickpeas are an excellent source of fiber and protein, while kale provides important vitamins and prebiotic fiber that feed healthy gut bacteria.

Ingredients:

- 1 cup cooked chickpeas
- 2 cups chopped kale
- 1 tablespoon tahini
- Juice of 1 lemon
- 1 tablespoon olive oil
- Salt and pepper to taste

Instructions:

- In a large bowl, combine the chickpeas and kale.
- In a small bowl, whisk together the tahini, lemon juice, olive oil, salt, and pepper.
- Pour the dressing over the salad and toss to combine.

Dinner Recipes

Dinner recipes focus on nutrient-dense meals that are anti-inflammatory and support gut healing. These recipes incorporate lean proteins, healthy fats, and a variety of vegetables to nourish your body while maintaining digestive health.

7. Roasted Salmon with Sweet Potatoes and Asparagus

This meal provides omega-3 fatty acids from salmon, which reduce inflammation, and fiber from sweet potatoes and asparagus to promote healthy digestion.

Ingredients:

- 2 salmon fillets
- 1 sweet potato, cubed
- 1 bunch asparagus
- 1 tablespoon olive oil
- Juice of 1 lemon
- Salt and pepper to taste

Instructions:

- Preheat your oven to 400°F (200°C).

- Toss the sweet potatoes in olive oil, salt, and pepper and spread them on a baking sheet. Roast for 20 minutes.
- Add the salmon fillets and asparagus to the baking sheet, drizzle with lemon juice and olive oil, and season with salt and pepper.
- Roast for another 12-15 minutes until the salmon is cooked through and the asparagus is tender.

8. Turmeric Chicken with Cauliflower Rice

Turmeric is a potent anti-inflammatory ingredient, and this recipe pairs it with chicken and cauliflower rice to create a light yet filling dinner that's easy on the digestive system.

Ingredients:

- 2 chicken breasts, diced
- 1 tablespoon olive oil
- 1 teaspoon turmeric
- 1 head cauliflower, grated into "rice"
- 1 garlic clove, minced
- Salt and pepper to taste

Instructions:

- Heat the olive oil in a pan and sauté the chicken with turmeric until cooked through.
- In a separate pan, sauté the cauliflower rice and garlic until tender. Season with salt and pepper.
- Serve the turmeric chicken over the cauliflower rice.

9. Zucchini Noodles with Pesto and Grilled Shrimp

This low-carb, gut-friendly meal is light yet full of flavor. The pesto is made from fresh basil and olive oil, while the grilled shrimp provides lean protein.

Ingredients:

- 2 zucchinis, spiralized into noodles
- 1/2 cup fresh basil leaves
- 1/4 cup olive oil
- 1 garlic clove
- 12 large shrimp, peeled and deveined
- Salt and pepper to taste

Instructions:

- Grill the shrimp until pink and cooked through.
- Blend the basil, olive oil, garlic, and salt in a food processor to make the pesto.
- Toss the zucchini noodles in the pesto and top with the grilled shrimp before serving.

Snacks and Sides

In between meals, it's important to have gut-friendly snacks on hand to keep you energized without causing digestive issues. These snacks are simple to prepare and full of prebiotic and probiotic ingredients that support gut health.

10. Apple Slices with Almond Butter and Flaxseeds

Ingredients:

- 1 apple, sliced
- 2 tablespoons almond butter
- 1 teaspoon ground flaxseeds

Instructions:

- Spread the almond butter on the apple slices.
- Sprinkle with flaxseeds for an extra fiber boost.
- 11. Greek Yogurt with Chia Seeds and Honey

Ingredients:

- 1 cup plain Greek yogurt
- 1 tablespoon chia seeds
- 1 teaspoon honey (optional)

Instructions:

- Mix the chia seeds into the Greek yogurt.
- Drizzle with honey if desired.

Fermented Food Recipes

Fermented foods provide a natural source of probiotics, which help maintain a healthy gut microbiome. These simple recipes for homemade fermented foods can be easily incorporated into your daily diet to keep your gut flora in balance.

12. Homemade Sauerkraut

Ingredients:

- 1 medium green cabbage, shredded
- 1 tablespoon sea salt

Instructions:

- Massage the salt into the shredded cabbage until it releases its juices.
- Pack the cabbage tightly into a clean glass jar, making sure it's submerged in its own liquid.
- Cover and let it ferment at room temperature for 1-4 weeks, checking occasionally.

- Store in the fridge once fermented.

13. Easy Kimchi

Ingredients:

- 1 medium napa cabbage, chopped
- 2 tablespoons sea salt
- 4 garlic cloves, minced
- 1 tablespoon ginger, minced
- 2 tablespoons chili flakes
- 2 tablespoons fish sauce (optional)

Instructions:

- Soak the cabbage in salted water for 2 hours. Drain and rinse.
- Combine garlic, ginger, chili flakes, and fish sauce with the cabbage and pack tightly into a glass jar.
- Let it ferment at room temperature for 3-7 days.
- Once fermented, store in the fridge.

Long-Term Gut Health Through Food

This Post-Cleanse Recipe Book offers a wide variety of gut-friendly meals designed to help you maintain the benefits of the 15-Day Herbal Gut Reset. By continuing to nourish your body with whole, nutrient-dense foods, probiotics, and prebiotics, you'll support long-term gut health, reduce inflammation, and improve digestion. These recipes are simple, delicious, and perfect for incorporating into your daily routine, ensuring that you continue to thrive on your journey toward optimal wellness.

Bonus 3: Guided Meditation Series for Gut Health

Guided Meditation Series for Gut Health: Harnessing the Gut-Brain Connection

Your digestive health isn't just influenced by the foods you eat—it's also deeply connected to your mental and emotional well-being. The **gut-brain connection,** a bidirectional communication network between the gut and the brain, plays a critical role in your digestive health. Stress, anxiety, and other emotional states can negatively impact digestion, leading to issues such as bloating, indigestion, and even gut inflammation.

The **Guided Meditation Series for Gut Health** is designed to help you manage stress, promote relaxation, and support the natural healing processes of your digestive system. By engaging in regular meditation, you can calm your nervous system, reduce inflammation, and create a healthy environment for your gut microbiome to thrive.

In this series, you'll find various guided meditations tailored to reduce stress and anxiety, enhance mindful eating, and encourage gut healing. These meditations are short, easy to follow, and designed to fit into your daily routine, helping you cultivate a greater sense of balance between your mind and body.

Why Meditation is Essential for Gut Health

The relationship between the brain and the gut is so powerful that many scientists refer to the gut as the "second brain." The **gut-brain axis** is a complex system that links the central nervous system (the brain and spinal cord) with the enteric nervous system (the gut's nervous system). This connection explains why emotional states like stress, worry, and fear can manifest as physical symptoms such as bloating, constipation, diarrhea, and gut inflammation.

Stress triggers the release of hormones such as **cortisol,** which can disrupt digestion, increase inflammation, and alter the balance of gut bacteria. Chronic stress can lead to long-term digestive problems, including irritable bowel syndrome (IBS) and leaky gut syndrome. Meditation helps counteract the effects of stress by activating the **parasympathetic nervous system**—also known as the "rest and digest" system—promoting relaxation, reducing cortisol levels, and enhancing digestion.

Benefits of Meditation for Gut Health:

- **Reduces stress and anxiety,** which are major contributors to digestive issues.
- **Activates the parasympathetic nervous system,** promoting digestion and nutrient absorption.
- **Decreases inflammation** in the gut, reducing the risk of gut dysbiosis and other digestive disorders.
- **Improves mindful eating,** helping you make healthier food choices and enhance digestion.
- **Balances the gut microbiome,** supporting the growth of beneficial bacteria.

Guided Meditation 1: Stress-Relief Meditation for Digestive Health (10 minutes)

Goal: Calm the nervous system and reduce the impact of stress on digestion.

Stress is one of the leading causes of digestive discomfort. This 10-minute meditation focuses on deep breathing and calming the mind, allowing the body to switch from the "fight-or-flight" response (which disrupts digestion) to the "rest-and-digest" mode, where digestion can occur smoothly.

How It Works:

- **Deep Breathing:** Deep, diaphragmatic breathing signals to the body that it is safe, activating the parasympathetic nervous system, which improves digestion and reduces inflammation.
- **Visualization:** This meditation incorporates guided imagery of the digestive system relaxing and functioning harmoniously, helping to reduce bloating, gas, and discomfort.

Instructions:

- Find a quiet, comfortable place to sit or lie down. Close your eyes and focus on your breathing.
- Inhale deeply through your nose for a count of 4, hold for a count of 4, and exhale slowly through your mouth for a count of 6.
- As you continue breathing deeply, visualize your stomach and intestines relaxing. Picture your digestive organs working smoothly and efficiently, free of tension and stress.
- Continue this deep, rhythmic breathing for 10 minutes, focusing on releasing any physical or emotional stress you may be holding in your gut.

When to Use: Practice this meditation when you feel stressed or overwhelmed, particularly before or after meals, to calm your mind and support digestion.

Guided Meditation 2: Mindful Eating Meditation (5 minutes)

Goal: Enhance the digestion process by eating mindfully and appreciating the nourishment food provides.

Mindful eating is about paying full attention to the experience of eating and drinking, both physically and emotionally. It involves noticing the colors, textures, flavors, and smells of your food and being aware of how your body responds to it. This 5-minute meditation can be done before or during meals to promote mindful eating, which in turn aids digestion and prevents overeating.

How It Works:

- **Sensory Awareness:** By paying attention to the sensory aspects of eating, you enhance the body's digestive response.

- **Slowing Down:** Eating slowly allows your digestive system to properly process food and absorb nutrients.
- **Gratitude:** Incorporating gratitude for the food you are about to eat helps cultivate a positive emotional state, which can improve digestion.

Instructions:

- Before eating, sit comfortably and take a moment to look at your food. Notice the colors, textures, and smells. Express gratitude for the nourishment your food provides.
- Close your eyes and take three deep breaths, inhaling deeply through your nose and exhaling slowly through your mouth. As you breathe, feel yourself becoming more present and grounded.
- As you take your first bite, chew slowly and thoroughly. Pay attention to the flavors and textures of the food. Notice how it feels in your mouth.
- Between bites, set your utensils down and take a deep breath. Pause to reflect on how the food is nourishing your body.
- Continue eating mindfully, savoring each bite and allowing your body to fully engage in the digestion process.

When to Use: Practice this meditation at the start of every meal to help improve digestion, prevent overeating, and enhance your overall relationship with food.

Guided Meditation 3: Gut Healing Visualization (15 minutes)

Goal: Promote gut healing through visualization, reduce inflammation, and encourage the restoration of the gut lining.

Visualization is a powerful tool that can help support physical healing by focusing the mind on positive imagery and intentions. In this 15-minute meditation, you will be guided to visualize your gut healing, reducing inflammation, and restoring balance to your digestive system. This meditation is especially beneficial for those experiencing digestive issues such as bloating, IBS, or leaky gut syndrome.

How It Works:

- **Healing Imagery:** Guided imagery helps your body relax and enhances the healing process by visualizing the gut in a state of harmony and balance.
- **Reducing Inflammation:** Visualization of inflammation being reduced can help lower the stress response, which contributes to gut inflammation.
- **Restoring the Gut Lining:** Visualizing the healing and strengthening of the gut lining promotes the repair of damaged tissues.

Instructions:

- Find a quiet place to sit or lie down. Close your eyes and take several deep, calming breaths.

- Begin by visualizing your digestive system. Picture your stomach, intestines, and gut working together in perfect harmony.
- Imagine a warm, soothing light entering your body, flowing through your digestive system, and healing any areas of inflammation or discomfort.
- As you breathe deeply, visualize this healing light restoring the lining of your gut, creating a protective barrier that strengthens your digestion and prevents harmful substances from entering your bloodstream.
- Continue to visualize your gut healing and functioning optimally. Feel a sense of calm and relaxation as your body naturally heals itself.
- Spend the last few minutes focusing on gratitude for your body's ability to heal and for the food that nourishes your gut.

When to Use: Practice this meditation during or after a period of digestive discomfort, or as part of your regular routine to promote ongoing gut healing.

Guided Meditation 4: Daily Affirmations for Digestive Wellness (5 minutes)

Goal: Cultivate positive thoughts and reinforce your commitment to gut health through daily affirmations.

Affirmations are positive statements that can help you overcome negative thoughts and self-doubt. Repeating affirmations regularly can shift your mindset and foster a more positive relationship with your body and health. This 5-minute meditation is designed to reinforce your commitment to digestive wellness through simple but powerful affirmations.

How It Works:

- **Positive Reinforcement:** Affirmations help shift your mental state and promote a healthier relationship with your body and food.
- **Self-Compassion:** By practicing affirmations, you cultivate self-compassion, which reduces stress and encourages better health outcomes.

Instructions:

- Sit comfortably, close your eyes, and take three deep breaths.
- As you breathe, repeat the following affirmations either silently or out loud:
  - ✓ "I trust my body to digest my food and nourish my health."
  - ✓ "My gut is strong, healthy, and capable of healing."
  - ✓ "I release any stress or tension that may affect my digestion."
  - ✓ "I am grateful for the food that nourishes my body and supports my well-being."
  - ✓ "Every day, my gut is becoming healthier and more balanced."
- As you repeat these affirmations, allow yourself to fully believe them. Feel a sense of calm and gratitude as you focus on the positive energy these affirmations bring to your body.
- Continue for 5 minutes, and then take one final deep breath before opening your eyes.

When to Use: Start your day with these affirmations to set a positive tone, or repeat them whenever you feel anxious or stressed about your digestion.

Guided Meditation 5: Sleep Meditation for Better Digestion (15 minutes)

Goal: Promote restful sleep, which is essential for digestive repair and overall gut health.

Sleep is one of the most important factors for maintaining gut health. During sleep, your body undergoes repair processes, including the healing of the gut lining and the regulation of the gut microbiome. This 15-minute sleep meditation helps you relax deeply and prepare for a restful night's sleep, promoting digestion and healing.

How It Works:

- Deep Relaxation: This meditation uses progressive muscle relaxation to calm the body and mind, promoting restful sleep and better digestion.
- Sleep-Induced Healing: By relaxing the body before sleep, this meditation encourages your digestive system to rest and repair during the night.

Instructions:

- Lie down in a comfortable position, close your eyes, and take several slow, deep breaths.
- Begin by focusing on your feet, noticing any tension there, and releasing it as you exhale. Slowly move your attention up your body, relaxing each area as you breathe.
- Once your entire body is relaxed, visualize yourself lying on a soft, warm surface. Imagine that with each breath, your digestive system is resting and healing.
- As you drift into sleep, repeat the affirmation, "I allow my body to rest and heal. My digestion is strong, and my gut is restoring itself."
- Let go of any lingering thoughts or worries, and allow yourself to fall into a deep, restful sleep.

When to Use: Practice this meditation before bed to enhance relaxation, improve sleep quality, and promote overnight digestive healing.

The Power of Meditation for Gut Health

The **Guided Meditation Series for Gut Health** offers a holistic approach to supporting your digestive system through mental and emotional wellness. By incorporating these meditations into your daily routine, you can reduce stress, enhance digestion, and promote long-term gut healing. The power of the gut-brain connection cannot be overstated—when your mind is calm and your emotions are balanced, your gut thrives. Use these meditations as a valuable tool in your journey toward lasting digestive health and overall well-being.

Bonus 4: Herbal Remedies Cheat Sheet

Herbal Remedies Cheat Sheet: Key Ingredients for Gut Health and How to Use Them

Herbal remedies have been used for centuries to support digestion, reduce inflammation, and promote overall gut health. Herbs can offer a natural and effective solution to many common digestive issues, from bloating and indigestion to gut inflammation and dysbiosis. This **Herbal Remedies Cheat Sheet** is a quick-reference guide to some of the most powerful digestive herbs, explaining how they work and providing easy ways to incorporate them into your daily routine.

By integrating these herbal remedies into your diet, you can continue to support your gut health long after completing the **15-Day Herbal Gut Reset.** These herbs will not only help maintain the balance of your gut microbiome but also promote smooth digestion and reduce inflammation, keeping your digestive system functioning optimally.

Why Herbal Remedies are Essential for Gut Health

Herbs are nature's medicine, offering potent healing properties without the side effects often associated with pharmaceuticals. When it comes to gut health, many herbs possess properties that soothe the digestive tract, reduce inflammation, support the liver's detoxifying function, and even promote the growth of beneficial bacteria in the gut.

Herbs can be categorized based on their digestive benefits:

- **Digestive Stimulants:** Herbs that increase bile production and promote digestion (e.g., dandelion, ginger).
- **Carminatives:** Herbs that reduce bloating and gas by relaxing the smooth muscles of the digestive system (e.g., fennel, peppermint).
- **Gut-Healing Herbs:** Herbs that soothe and repair the gut lining (e.g., licorice root, marshmallow root).
- **Anti-Inflammatory Herbs:** Herbs that reduce inflammation throughout the gut (e.g., turmeric, chamomile).

1. Ginger: The Warming Digestive Aid

How it Works: Ginger is one of the most well-known herbs for supporting digestion. It has powerful anti-inflammatory and antioxidant properties that help reduce gut inflammation, improve gastric motility, and ease nausea and indigestion. Ginger contains compounds called **gingerols** and **shogaols,** which stimulate digestive enzymes and improve the breakdown of food.

Benefits:

- Eases nausea and vomiting
- Reduces bloating and indigestion
- Stimulates digestion and promotes gut motility

How to Use:

- **Ginger Tea:** Simmer a 1-inch piece of fresh ginger in boiling water for 10 minutes. Add honey or lemon for taste and drink before meals to support digestion.
- **Grated Ginger:** Add freshly grated ginger to stir-fries, soups, or smoothies.
- **Ginger Supplements:** Take in capsule form, especially if you experience frequent nausea or indigestion.

2. Dandelion Root: The Liver Detoxifier

How it Works: Dandelion root is a powerful digestive herb that supports liver health and bile production. Bile is essential for breaking down fats and aiding in nutrient absorption. Dandelion root also acts as a gentle diuretic, helping to flush out toxins and support the kidneys in detoxification. It's especially beneficial for individuals with sluggish digestion or those looking to detoxify the liver.

Benefits:

- Stimulates bile production, aiding in fat digestion
- Supports liver detoxification and kidney function
- Helps relieve constipation and water retention

How to Use:

- **Dandelion Root Tea:** Simmer 1 tablespoon of dried dandelion root in boiling water for 10-15 minutes. Drink daily, especially after meals to support digestion and liver detox.
- **Dandelion Salads:** Use fresh dandelion greens in salads for a nutrient boost.
- **Supplements:** Dandelion root is available in capsule or tincture form for those who prefer a more concentrated dose.

3. Peppermint: The Carminative Antispasmodic

How it Works: Peppermint is known for its antispasmodic properties, meaning it helps to relax the smooth muscles in the digestive tract. This makes it highly effective in reducing bloating, gas, and abdominal cramps. Peppermint also promotes bile flow, which aids in fat digestion, and it can be particularly helpful for those with irritable bowel syndrome (IBS) or frequent indigestion.

Benefits:

- Reduces bloating, gas, and abdominal discomfort
- Relieves symptoms of IBS
- Supports bile flow for better fat digestion

How to Use:

- **Peppermint Tea:** Steep 1 teaspoon of dried peppermint leaves in hot water for 5-10 minutes. Drink after meals to prevent bloating and gas.

- **Peppermint Oil Capsules:** These are particularly effective for those with IBS. They deliver the benefits of peppermint directly to the intestines.
- **Fresh Peppermint:** Add fresh peppermint leaves to salads, fruit bowls, or as a garnish for beverages.

4. Fennel: The Bloat Buster

How it Works: Fennel seeds are a traditional remedy for bloating and indigestion. They act as a carminative, which helps relieve gas and relaxes the muscles in the digestive tract. Fennel also has mild anti-inflammatory properties and can stimulate the production of digestive enzymes, making it easier for the body to break down food.

Benefits:

- Relieves bloating, gas, and indigestion
- Promotes the secretion of digestive enzymes
- Helps soothe spasms in the digestive tract

How to Use:

- **Fennel Seed Tea:** Crush 1 teaspoon of fennel seeds and steep them in boiling water for 5-10 minutes. Drink after meals to reduce bloating and gas.
- **Chew Fennel Seeds:** After a meal, chew on a few fennel seeds to freshen your breath and aid digestion.
- **Add to Cooking:** Incorporate fennel seeds into your cooking, especially in soups and stews for added digestive support.

5. Licorice Root: The Gut Healer

How it Works: Licorice root is known for its soothing and anti-inflammatory properties, particularly in healing the gut lining. It stimulates mucus production, which protects the stomach and intestines from irritation. This makes it especially helpful for conditions like **leaky gut syndrome, acid reflux,** and **ulcers.** Look for **deglycyrrhizinated licorice (DGL),** as this form removes the compound glycyrrhizin, which can raise blood pressure in large amounts.

Benefits:

- Soothes and repairs the gut lining
- Reduces inflammation in the digestive tract
- Helps relieve symptoms of heartburn and acid reflux

How to Use:

- **Licorice Root Tea:** Steep 1 teaspoon of dried licorice root in hot water for 10 minutes. Drink 1-2 cups daily to soothe the gut and promote healing.

- **DGL Supplements:** For those with acid reflux or ulcers, DGL supplements are available in chewable tablets that can be taken before meals.
- **Add to Smoothies:** Use powdered licorice root in smoothies or juices for an easy digestive boost.

6. Turmeric: The Anti-Inflammatory Powerhouse

How it Works: Turmeric is one of the most potent anti-inflammatory herbs, known for its active compound **curcumin.** It reduces inflammation throughout the body, including in the digestive tract. Turmeric supports gut health by lowering inflammation in the gut lining, preventing and treating conditions like **IBS, Crohn's disease,** and **ulcerative colitis.** It also supports liver function, aiding in the detoxification process.

Benefits:

- Reduces inflammation in the gut
- Supports liver detoxification
- May help prevent and treat IBS, Crohn's, and colitis

How to Use:

- **Golden Milk:** Mix 1 teaspoon of turmeric powder with warm almond milk, a pinch of black pepper, and a teaspoon of honey for a soothing anti-inflammatory drink.
- **Turmeric Capsules:** Take curcumin supplements to boost your daily intake, particularly if you have chronic inflammation.
- **Add to Cooking:** Use turmeric in soups, stews, curries, or even scrambled eggs to add an anti-inflammatory punch to your meals.

7. Chamomile: The Soothing Digestive Tonic

How it Works: Chamomile is a gentle herb with calming and anti-inflammatory properties that soothe the digestive tract. It helps relieve indigestion, bloating, and cramping, while also promoting relaxation and reducing stress—two factors that are crucial for gut health. Chamomile can also help ease symptoms of gastritis, acid reflux, and IBS by calming the gut lining.

Benefits:

- Reduces bloating and cramping
- Soothes inflammation in the gut
- Relieves symptoms of acid reflux and IBS

How to Use:

- **Chamomile Tea:** Steep 1 tablespoon of dried chamomile flowers in hot water for 5-10 minutes. Drink 1-2 cups daily, especially before bed to aid digestion and promote restful sleep.
- **Chamomile Tincture:** Use a few drops of chamomile tincture in water or tea for a more concentrated dose.

- **Add to Baths:** Chamomile-infused baths can promote relaxation and reduce overall stress, which positively impacts gut health.

8. Marshmallow Root: The Gut Protector

How it Works: Marshmallow root has mucilage properties, meaning it creates a protective layer of mucus along the gut lining. This makes it particularly useful for soothing irritation caused by conditions like leaky gut, gastritis, and ulcers. Marshmallow root helps repair damaged tissues in the gut and protects against further irritation from stomach acid.

Benefits:

- Soothes and protects the gut lining
- Reduces inflammation and irritation in the digestive tract
- Helps heal conditions like leaky gut and ulcers

How to Use:

- **Marshmallow Root Tea:** Steep 1 tablespoon of dried marshmallow root in cold water for at least 4 hours, then strain and drink. This "cold infusion" preserves the mucilage properties of the root.
- **Powdered Marshmallow Root:** Add powdered marshmallow root to smoothies or water to help soothe the digestive tract.
- **Supplements:** Take marshmallow root in capsule form to support long-term gut healing.

9. Milk Thistle: The Liver Protector

How it Works: Milk thistle is primarily known for its liver-supporting properties, but since the liver plays a key role in digestion, milk thistle indirectly supports gut health. It helps detoxify the liver, promotes bile production, and protects the liver from damage caused by toxins, alcohol, and fatty foods. Bile production is critical for breaking down fats and aiding in digestion.

Benefits:

- Supports liver detoxification and bile production
- Protects the liver from toxins
- Aids in fat digestion and nutrient absorption

How to Use:

- **Milk Thistle Tea:** Steep 1 teaspoon of crushed milk thistle seeds in boiling water for 10 minutes. Drink daily to support liver health.
- **Milk Thistle Capsules:** For a concentrated dose, take milk thistle supplements to promote liver detoxification and overall digestive support.
- **Add to Smoothies:** Use powdered milk thistle in smoothies for an easy way to integrate it into your diet.

How to Incorporate Herbs into Your Daily Routine
The best way to experience the full benefits of these herbs is to incorporate them into your daily routine. Here are some practical ways to do this:

- **Start Your Day with Herbal Teas:** Begin your day with a gut-soothing tea, such as ginger, peppermint, or chamomile, to kickstart digestion and reduce bloating.
- **Add Herbs to Your Cooking:** Use fresh or dried herbs like turmeric, ginger, and fennel in your cooking to support digestion with every meal.
- **Use Herbal Supplements:** For convenience, consider herbal supplements in capsule, tincture, or powder form to ensure you get the necessary therapeutic doses of these powerful herbs.
- **Combine Herbs in Smoothies:** Add powdered or fresh herbs like ginger, licorice root, or turmeric to your morning smoothies for a daily gut health boost.

Harnessing the Power of Herbs for Gut Health
This **Herbal Remedies Cheat Sheet** is your quick-reference guide to some of the most potent digestive herbs, each offering unique benefits for gut health. Whether you're looking to soothe inflammation, reduce bloating, or promote liver detoxification, these herbs can be powerful allies in maintaining your digestive wellness. By incorporating these herbs into your daily routine, you can continue to support your gut health naturally, long after completing the **15-Day Herbal Gut Reset.**

Bonus 5: 15-Day Accountability Tracker
15-Day Accountability Tracker: Staying on Track with Your Gut Health Journey

The **15-Day Herbal Gut Reset** is a transformative experience designed to reset your digestive health and restore balance to your gut microbiome. While the detox plan provides the foundation for success, staying on track and maintaining your motivation can be challenging, especially as you adjust your diet and habits. The **15-Day Accountability Tracker** is a powerful tool that helps you monitor your progress, hold yourself accountable, and celebrate your victories along the way.

This tracker is not just about following the plan—it's about reflecting on your journey, tracking daily behaviors that support gut health, and recognizing the positive changes happening in your body. By keeping a daily log of your meals, hydration, herbal teas, physical activity, detox symptoms, and non-scale victories (NSVs), you'll have a clear record of your accomplishments and challenges. This tracker will help you stay motivated, maintain consistency, and ultimately achieve long-term success in improving your digestive health.

Why Use a 15-Day Accountability Tracker?
Accountability is one of the key factors in achieving any health goal, and the **15-Day Herbal Gut Reset** is no exception. By tracking your daily actions, you'll be more mindful of the choices you make, more aware of your progress, and better equipped to adjust when challenges arise. The accountability tracker is designed to keep you on course throughout the detox, but its benefits go beyond the 15-day period. It will also help you develop sustainable habits that will continue to support your gut health after the reset is complete.

Key Benefits of Using the Accountability Tracker:

- **Daily Tracking:** Provides structure by allowing you to track your meals, hydration, herbal teas, physical activity, and symptoms every day.
- **Reflection and Awareness:** Prompts you to reflect on how your body feels, helping you recognize patterns and make adjustments as needed.
- **Motivation:** Encourages you to stay consistent and committed by celebrating small wins, such as improved digestion or increased energy.
- **Non-Scale Victories:** Emphasizes health improvements that go beyond weight loss, such as reduced bloating, clearer skin, or better sleep.
- **Long-Term Habit Formation:** By tracking your progress, you'll be more likely to develop sustainable habits that support your gut health well after the 15 days are over.

Components of the 15-Day Accountability Tracker

The **15-Day Accountability Tracker** includes various sections that cover all aspects of the gut reset process, ensuring that you're logging the most important elements of your detox journey. Below is a detailed breakdown of each section and how to use it.

1. Daily Meal Tracker

Goal: Track your meals to ensure you are following the gut-friendly guidelines of the detox, incorporating whole foods, fiber-rich vegetables, and anti-inflammatory ingredients. This section also helps you reflect on how your meals make you feel, so you can identify foods that work well for your digestion and those that may cause discomfort.

How to Use:

- **Record Each Meal:** Log your breakfast, lunch, dinner, and snacks every day. Be specific about the ingredients and portion sizes. For example, "Breakfast: Smoothie with spinach, chia seeds, banana, and almond milk" or "Lunch: Quinoa salad with kale, avocado, and olive oil dressing."
- **Note Food Sensitivities:** If you notice any digestive discomfort after certain meals (e.g., bloating, gas, or cramping), write it down. This will help you identify any potential food sensitivities or triggers.
- **Reflect on Satisfaction:** After each meal, reflect on how satisfied you feel. Did the meal leave you feeling energized or sluggish? Full or still hungry? This reflection will help you adjust portion sizes or food choices if needed.

Example Entry:

- **Breakfast:** Chia pudding with almond milk, topped with blueberries and a drizzle of honey.
- **Lunch:** Grilled chicken salad with spinach, avocado, and lemon-tahini dressing.
- **Dinner:** Roasted vegetables (sweet potatoes, zucchini, and carrots) with quinoa and a turmeric dressing.
- **Snack:** Apple slices with almond butter.
- **Notes:** Felt bloated after lunch—will try reducing the portion size of avocado tomorrow.

2. Hydration and Herbal Tea Tracker

Goal: Hydration is crucial for digestive health and detoxification. The hydration and herbal tea tracker ensures you're drinking enough water and detox-supporting herbal teas to stay hydrated and promote digestion.

How to Use:

- **Water Intake:** Record how many glasses of water you drink each day. Aim for at least 8-10 glasses of water per day, but adjust based on your body's needs and activity level.
- **Herbal Teas:** Log any herbal teas you drink, such as ginger, peppermint, or dandelion root tea. These teas support digestion, reduce bloating, and aid in liver detoxification.

Example Entry:

- **Water:** 8 glasses of water today.
- **Herbal Tea:** 1 cup of ginger tea before breakfast, 1 cup of peppermint tea after lunch.
- **Notes:** Felt more energized today after increasing water intake.

3. Physical Activity and Movement Log

Goal: Physical activity stimulates digestion and supports detoxification by promoting gut motility and reducing stress. This section allows you to track your daily movement, whether it's a structured workout or gentle exercises like walking or yoga.

How to Use:

- **Record Your Exercise:** Log any physical activity you do each day. This can include workouts (e.g., strength training, cardio, yoga) or gentle movement like walking or stretching.
- **Reflect on How You Feel:** After each workout, note how your body feels. Do you notice improved digestion after moving your body? Are you feeling more energetic or less bloated after exercise?

Example Entry:

- **Activity:** 30-minute walk in the morning, 20 minutes of yoga in the evening.
- **Notes:** Felt less bloated and more energized after the walk. Yoga helped me relax before bed.

4. Detox Symptoms Journal

Goal: The detox process can bring about various symptoms as your body adjusts to the elimination of processed foods and toxins. The detox symptoms journal allows you to monitor any physical or emotional symptoms you experience throughout the 15 days.

How to Use:

- **Track Symptoms:** Each day, note any detox symptoms you experience, such as headaches, fatigue, irritability, digestive discomfort, or cravings. These symptoms are common during the first few days of the detox but should improve as your body adjusts.
- **Note Emotional Changes:** Detoxing can also affect your mood and emotions. Record any emotional shifts, such as feeling more relaxed, anxious, or motivated.
- **Identify Patterns:** By tracking symptoms daily, you may notice patterns, such as feeling more energized on days when you drink more water or fewer symptoms when you get enough sleep.

Example Entry:

- **Symptoms:** Mild headache in the afternoon, feeling more tired than usual. Some bloating after dinner.
- **Emotional Changes:** Felt more irritable today, especially in the morning.
- **Notes:** Increased water intake helped reduce the headache.

5. Non-Scale Victories (NSVs) Log

Goal: The **Non-Scale Victories (NSVs)** section encourages you to focus on positive changes in your body and health that aren't related to weight. This helps keep you motivated and reinforces the fact that the cleanse is about overall wellness, not just numbers on a scale.

How to Use:

- **Record Daily NSVs:** Each day, note any non-scale victories you experience. These can include improved digestion (less bloating, regular bowel movements), increased energy, clearer skin, better sleep, reduced cravings, or improved mood.
- **Celebrate Small Wins:** Every improvement, no matter how small, is a victory. By celebrating these wins, you'll stay motivated and reinforce the positive impact the detox is having on your health.

Example Entry:

- **NSVs Today:** Woke up feeling more rested and less bloated. My skin looks clearer, and I had more energy throughout the day.
- **Notes:** I'm feeling more in control of my food choices and less tempted to snack on unhealthy foods.

6. Weekly Reflection

Goal: At the end of each week, reflect on your overall progress, challenges, and how you're feeling. This weekly reflection helps you take stock of the bigger picture and make any necessary adjustments for the upcoming week.

How to Use:

- **Reflect on Progress:** Write about the positive changes you've experienced in the past week. What improvements have you noticed in your digestion, energy, mood, or overall well-being?
- **Identify Challenges:** Reflect on any challenges or obstacles you faced. Were there any days you found it difficult to stay on track? How did you overcome these challenges?
- **Set Goals for the Next Week:** Based on your reflection, set goals for the upcoming week. These could include increasing your water intake, getting more sleep, or focusing on mindful eating.

Example Entry:

- **Week 1 Reflection:** This week, I noticed a big improvement in my energy levels and digestion. My bloating has gone down, and I feel more in control of my food choices. The biggest challenge was dealing with cravings in the evening, but drinking herbal tea helped. For next week, I want to focus on getting more sleep and continuing to drink enough water.

Tips for Success with the Accountability Tracker

Here are a few tips to help you get the most out of your **15-Day Accountability Tracker:**

- **Be Honest:** This tracker is for your benefit, so be honest with yourself about your progress, challenges, and habits. If you slip up or have a difficult day, use it as an opportunity to reflect and adjust, rather than judging yourself.
- **Use the Tracker Daily:** Consistency is key. Make it a habit to fill out the tracker at the same time every day, whether in the morning or before bed.
- **Review Your Progress Regularly:** At the end of each week, take time to review your entries and look for patterns. What's working well? What areas need improvement? Use these insights to make adjustments for the following week.
- **Celebrate Your Wins:** Whether it's improved digestion, clearer skin, or increased energy, celebrate every victory. Recognizing your progress is a powerful motivator to keep going.
- **Make Adjustments as Needed:** If you notice that certain foods or habits are causing discomfort, use the tracker to make adjustments. This process is about learning what works best for your body and making changes that support long-term gut health.

Empowering Your Gut Health Journey

The **15-Day Accountability Tracker** is more than just a tool for keeping track of your meals and hydration—it's a powerful resource that helps you stay mindful, reflect on your progress, and celebrate your achievements throughout the **15-Day Herbal Gut Reset.** By using this tracker, you'll develop a deeper awareness of how your body responds to the detox process and gain valuable insights into your digestive health.

This tracker empowers you to take charge of your health, stay accountable to your goals, and make lasting changes that support long-term gut health. Whether you're celebrating non-scale victories, adjusting your meals based on how you feel, or reflecting on your weekly progress, this accountability tracker will keep you motivated and on track to achieve the vibrant, healthy life you deserve.

References

Gibson, G. R., & Roberfroid, M. B. (2010). *Dietary modulation of the human colonic microbiota: Introducing the concept of prebiotics.* Journal of Nutrition, 125(6), 1401-1412.

Bäckhed, F., Ley, R. E., Sonnenburg, J. L., Peterson, D. A., & Gordon, J. I. (2005). *Host-bacterial mutualism in the human intestine. Science,* 307(5717), 1915-1920.

Turnbaugh, P. J., Ley, R. E., Hamady, M., Fraser-Liggett, C. M., Knight, R., & Gordon, J. I. (2007). *The human microbiome project. Nature,* 449(7164), 804-810.

Cummings, J. H., & Macfarlane, G. T. (2002). *Gastrointestinal effects of prebiotics. British Journal of Nutrition,* 87(S2), S145-S151.

Vrieze, A., Van Nood, E., Holleman, F., Salojärvi, J., Kootte, R. S., & Bartelsman, J. F. W. M. (2012). *Transfer of intestinal microbiota from lean donors increases insulin sensitivity in individuals with metabolic syndrome. Gastroenterology,* 143(4), 913-916.

Sonnenburg, J. L., & Bäckhed, F. (2016). *Diet-microbiota interactions as moderators of human metabolism.* Nature, 535(7610), 56-64.

Mayer, E. A., & Tillisch, K. (2011). *The brain-gut axis in abdominal pain syndromes. Annual Review of Medicine,* 62(1), 381-396.

Klement, R. J., & Pazienza, V. (2019). *Impact of different types of fasting on the gut microbiota and immune system. Current Opinion in Clinical Nutrition and Metabolic Care,* 22(6), 401-407.

Sokol, H., & Seksik, P. (2010). *The role of intestinal microbiota in chronic inflammatory diseases. Clinical Reviews in Allergy & Immunology,* 38(3), 313-321.

Hutkins, R. W., & Krumbeck, J. A. (2012). *Gut microbiota and its implications for health and disease. Annual Review of Food Science and Technology,* 3, 71-93.